ARTHRITIS, RHEUMATISM and OSTEOPOROSIS

AN EFFECTIVE PROGRAM FOR CORRECTION THROUGH NUTRITION

By Bernard Jensen, Ph.D.

THE INFORMATION PRESENTED HERE WAS GATHERED DURING OVER 50 YEARS OF SANITARIUM EXPERIENCE, WORKING WITH DIET, EXERCISE AND THE NATURAL HEALING ART TO BRING PATIENTS TO A RIGHT WAY OF LIVING, A PAIN-FREE LIFE WITH NO UNDESIRABLE SIDE EFFECTS, USING THE LATEST, MOST UP-TO-DATE NUTRITIONAL RESEARCH AVAILABLE.

Published by
Bernard Jensen Enterprises
24360 Old Wagon Road
Escondido, California 92027

This book is intended for use as an information source. It is not intended as advice for self-diagnosis or a prescription for self treatment. It is hoped that the information contained herein will stimulate thought and encourage the adoption of a beneficial lifestyle.

COVER: A thermograph of arthritic hands, showing the heat concentrated in the feverish, inflamed areas. The inflammation causes minerals to be consumed at an abnormal rate. Modern photography has developed techniques for taking photos showing concentration of heat in areas of the body. The ancient Greeks anticipated thermographic techniques by placing mud packs on their patients. The parts that dried first revealed the most feverish areas of the body and the location of the greatest amount of heat.

First Edition

BERNARD JENSEN, Publisher
Route 1, Box 52
Escondido, CA 92025

ISBN 0-932615-03-1

Introduction

This book will be a great help to anyone with arthritis, other rheumatoid conditions or osteoporosis. If a complete solution to rheumatoid diseases is ever found, I believe it will be along the lines of the program I am presenting here, which is based on over 50 years of private sanitarium practice. This book is to teach you to take care of your problems, rather than giving you temporary relief. Take care of your problems that are yet to come. Let us prevent more and cure less. Let us live a good lifestyle so we need less treatments.

So many people are taking gold shots, injections, vaccinations and nostrums for relief—only relief. My program offers correction, a method of bringing in new tissue through evolved living, if the disease is not too far advanced.

Arthritis may take many years to reach the degenerative stage, and it is possible to wait too long before starting a corrective program. If the condition is not too advanced, my program should help. I have had excellent success in dissolving calcium deposits and spurs from those who have had osteoarthritis.

In fact, Dr. Waterson, a medical doctor from Scottsdale, Arizona, used to visit my Ranch and watch how my program of nutrition and exercise affected people with different diseases. Once he showed me six photographs of a man's knee, taken over a year and a half, showing the progressive reduction of a large calcium spur down to nothing. Calcium deposits can be reversed. Dr. Waterson used only my methods with this patient.

I have also worked with Dr. Henry G. Bieler of Pasadena, author of *Food Is Your Best Medicine,* showing him my nutritional program. I worked with him on over 500 cases, with many wonderful results, including arthritis cases. His book was based on his success in treating various rheumatoid problems with injections and oral administration of hydrochloric acid. His success was due to improvement of protein digestion. Many people with rheumatoid problems would benefit from taking digestive aid tablets and foods high in sodium. The stomach wall uses a good deal of sodium in the process of digestion. When sodium becomes depleted, it must be replaced for proper digestion of protein.

In my estimation, over 50 percent of the people in this country have some form of rheumatoid disturbance, ranging from slight pain and stiffness in the morning to the most degenerative stages. This includes people with nodules on the joints, bone spurs and joint problems of all kinds. I am including osteoporosis (calcium loss from the bones) because it is a calcium imbalance problem, even though it is not a rheumatoid condition. There are millions of people in this country who have these conditions, and my program of diet, exercise and nutritional supplements could help many of them, although I cannot say it will help all.

The causes of rheumatoid conditions are many. Trauma, fatigue, genetic disposition, sodium deficiency, metabolic disorders, poor food habits, junk food, high-stress jobs or lifestyles, drug side effects, food allergies, chemicalized drinking water, excessive perspiration (sodium loss), glandular imbalance, climate, excessive use of meat and many other things can contribute to the development of rheumatoid problems.

Digestive problems may lead to or result from rheumatoid conditions, but they nearly always go together. Once the digestive difficulties begin, the body is unable to assimilate all the nutrients it needs. A high percentage of my patients are deficient in hydrochloric acid, needed to digest proteins properly. When we realize that most of our calcium is from proteins, we can see the problem. We must work to improve digestion if we are to take care of rheumatoid problems.

Excess table salt, which is the wrong kind of sodium, contributes to hardening of the arteries, and I believe it contributes to joint troubles as well. I advise cutting it out of the diet, or at least, cutting down on the use of it as much as possible.

The people of the United States are on a calcium craze now. Television advertising and magazine ads are loaded with new products claiming to be the solution to the problem of calcium deficiency. Osteoporosis and other types of calcium-imbalance problems, such as osteoarthritis and rheumatoid arthritis, are suddenly in the forefront of the news.

How real is the problem? And, how realistic are the solutions proposed by advertisers?

In over 50 years of sanitarium practice, I have taken care of thousands of cases of arthritis, and I can tell you, the problem is very real. And the reason I have written this book is because I have found a very real and lasting answer.

Recent surveys show that American women, aged 16 to 50, are getting less than 70% of the recommended daily allowance of calcium, which is 1000 mg. An advertisement by Kraft, the well-known U.S. manufacturer of processed cheese, claims that 50% of American children are getting less than their recommended daily allowance of calcium. They are urging parents to give their children more cheese. I believe these reports. I believe that a high percentage of Americans do not get enough calcium—or at least not enough of the right kind of calcium. But, I don't believe that taking some highly advertised calcium supplement will necessarily help.

First of all, I want you to notice that most of the remedies offered for the pain and stiffness of arthritis are *for relief only*. They don't pretend to get at the *cause* of the problem. They don't offer correction.

Most people with arthritis or other painful rheumatic conditions just want to get rid of the pain. They don't realize these are unseen causes inside the body that are producing the pain. I don't care how much Advil, Tylenol or aspirin you take, the pain will always return until you make up your mind to go after the cause of the problem and get rid of it. Most people and their doctors look at pain as a localized thing, and that's the way they treat it. I believe that 90% of our aches and pains are reflex pain from some other part of the body. You can't treat the local site of pain, which is a symptom only, and get rid of its deeper cause in some other part of the body.

Are drugs the answer? In two recent experiments, one at the University of California's San Diego Medical Center and the other at the University of Kansas Arthritis Center, new drugs were tested. Improvement was found with both drugs, although side effects were found for one, and after it was stopped, symptoms became worse than ever. No doubt the other has side effects, too—because all drugs have side effects. The problem with drugs is that they disturb the body chemistry, cause dangerous side effects and leave toxic residues in the body. Drugs tend to relieve symptoms without getting at the underlying cause, and, although drugs can alter the body chemistry, they cannot rebuild tissue, they cannot replace old tissue with new, which is what is required for complete healing to take place.

After age 50, when rheumatic conditions begin to appear in the majority of those who get them, there is 20% lowered function in all parts of the body, due to aging. Elimination of wastes is retarded. The skin becomes dry. Thyroid function is lower, reducing glandular function throughout the body and lowering the metabolism. To develop a realistic program for taking care of arthritis and other rheumatic conditions, we need to recognize what is going on in the whole body and take care of everything—toxic settlements, mineral deficiencies and a diminished immunity.

The wholistic approach to taking care of a disease or condition is to build up the health of the whole body until the body is strong enough to throw off the problem. In the case of rheumatic conditions, we need to use iodine for the thyroid, exercise and hawthorn berry tea for the circulation, sufficient liquid intake and KB-11 tea to take care of the kidneys, fresh vegetables and fruits to provide enough natural fiber to increase bowel elimination, foods high in calcium, sodium and potassium to neutralize excess body acids, vitamin D to help with calcium assimilation, and a proper diet to meet all nutrient needs and correct deficiencies. This is just an idea of a few things to take care of a few problems that exist. Each person is different, having different vital organ problems that would need other types of corrective measures. This is a wholistic approach, the way of working with nature instead of trying to find shortcuts by man's way.

We need to understand that every gland, organ and tissue in the body affects every other part of the body. We live in an acid-producing country where the pressures of our jobs, urban living and relationships produce a lot of nerve acids. We have to live with environmental pollution, the problems of a high-speed technological society, financial troubles and devitalized, processed foods that do not nourish our bodies properly.

The problem with most commercially-produced calcium supplements is that they are not balanced for human assimilation. Calcium must be balanced with magnesium, and if there is too much or too little of one or the other, it cannot be used properly by the body. There must be enough vitamin D in the body to help assimilate calcium. Without exercise, our bodies can't take in sufficient calcium as needed, even if we take calcium pills with three times the recommended daily allowance. It is excreted from the body instead.

Calcium supplements alone are not the answer in calcium deficiency problems. We need to use high calcium foods, instead. Only nature combines calcium with the right balance of other minerals, enzymes and vitamins.

On the other hand, many people who are developing enlarged joints and calcium spurs feel they are caused by taking too much calcium. This is not usually the case. The trouble is usually calcium-sodium imbalance in the body, resulting in calcium coming out of solution in the blood and depositing in the joints. We still need calcium, but we need to have a diet high in natural sodium foods at the same time.

There are other problems. A University of Washington study showed that caffeine, as found in coffee, tea, chocolate and most soft drinks, increases calcium loss in the body by double. Sugar leaches calcium out of the body. By the way, these so-called foods are very acid forming. You don't need more acid foods of this kind to add to the rheumatic acid you already have.

Drinking more milk has been proposed as a solution to calcium imbalance in arthritis and osteoporosis, and Dale Alexander, author of *Arthritis and Common Sense,* has had good results giving milk with a little cod liver oil added to many people with arthritis. This is a good remedy for some people, but I believe we need to take a larger view of the problem and consider the needs of the whole body. Milk, for example, will not take care of the sodium deficiency which is often the cause of calcium imbalance in the body. The truth is, the average American has 25% milk products in his diet, according to USDA figures, and this is not solving the calcium imbalance problem for most people.

Dr. John Ott found a link between the ultraviolet in sunlight and arthritis. Because most people work indoors most of the time, they don't get enough ultraviolet from artificial light, especially fluorescent lights. Window glass and the glasses most people wear filter out 85% of the ultraviolet, and the eyes are unable to take in this light. Ott's arthritis disappeared after he broke his glasses while on vacation in Florida, and he believes it is very important that we take in ultraviolet through the eyes every day. It doesn't have to be direct sunlight. We still get ultraviolet light when we are outside in the shade from reflections. I recommend plastic lenses over glass lenses in glasses, because they let in 85% of the ultraviolet, instead of only 15% as regular glass lenses do.

Glandular imbalances can lead to rheumatic conditions. The thyroid gland not only influences every other endocrine gland in the body, but regulates the body's metabolism and blood levels of calcium. So, when the thyroid is underactive, the whole body's energy supply and chemical balance is affected.

"You are as young as your glands," they say. Keeping the glands balanced will help keep joints young and limber. I have found that those with an active, enjoyable sex life have less trouble with arthritis than those who do not. I'm not saying sex is necessary for everyone, but there can be such a thing as subnormal sexuality when the body has not been kept up right. There is definitely a relationship between the health of the glands and the joints.

Rheumatic conditions and arthritis may be caused by drug residues or side effects from drugs taken in the past. They may be caused by an inadequate diet, by too many fad diets, or by junk foods. Pollution, food allergies and lack of exercise can contribute to arthritis.

I have found out that certain natural laws have to be followed to stay in good health and avoid disease. When we violate these laws, we invite problems, and over a long period of time, the problem can develop into a disease. To get rid of the disease and bring the body back to good health, we have to bring in new tissue to replace the old, and this can only be done through proper foods. This is correction, not relief. This is a wholistic health program leading to a permanent change.

Many therapies will help rheumatoid conditions. Reflexology, water treatments, massage, epsom salt baths and herbs, but none of them can bring correction of the cause unless proper nutrition is used with it. None can do much good unless you change the lifestyle habits that are contributing to your troubles. We have to stop breaking down before we can build up tissue and repair past damage.

Relief measures offered by shots and drugs cannot cure you. They are only for temporary relief of pain. Even if hospitals use one brand of pain relief drug over another doesn't mean it is better. Taking these pain relievers only puts off the real internal problem to a later date to be cared for—and which may be serious to correct because you didn't take care of the cause. You took care of the symptom only.

Pain relief will also come, in many cases, from following my program, although it may take longer. Your condition did not develop overnight, and nature cannot cure you overnight. It will take time.

A warm climate favors getting rid of rheumatoid conditions. Symptoms are usually relieved. If you live where winters are cold, go south in the winter if you can. Three seasons in a row of warm weather would build up your immune system and health so you could overcome your problems better. It usually takes a year to see substantial progress in working with any chronic condition.

Exercise is another necessary ingredient of taking care of rheumatoid conditions. The lymphatic system cannot function properly without exercise, and it is the lymph that carries nutrients into the joints and carries out the wastes, where blood cannot enter. Lymph works like a gas, getting into places the blood can't reach. An active lymph system is needed to have youthful joints. Only the lymph can get sodium into many of the joints. And, by the way, the lymph fluid is a high sodium fluid.

We need to perspire to get rid of toxic wastes, but we also need to replace the loss of sodium that comes from perspiring. Commercial soft drinks are usually high in caffeine, phosphorus and sugar, all of which leach calcium from the body. Don't use them. After perspiring heavily, take fruit juice, a vegetable broth drink or a whey drink. We have to constantly replace sodium lost by the body, especially if we have jobs requiring hard manual labor or long periods of intense physical activity, such as in professional athletics, etc.

Several studies support my long-held view that dietary factors are important in bringing about the development of arthritis and other rheumatoid conditions. A study by Dr. W.A. Hennings in England showed that incompletely broken-down proteins in the bloodstream could be traced to gluten-containing products, such as wheat, in the diet. These incomplete proteins tend to aggravate the inflammation of arthritis. Since 29% of the average American diet comes from wheat, this creates a favorable environment for arthritis.

Similarly, food allergies are belived to aggravate symptoms of arthritis, or even cause it in some cases, as described in a 1983 article in the *Journal of the International Academy of Preventive Medicine.* I believe food alergies may often be generated by abnormal chemical reactions in the body triggered by refined foods or chemicalized foods with unnatural additives. The body is designed to digest and assimilate foods as made by nature, and man's tampering with foods has not always been to our benefit.

Most of my patients lack adequate hydrochloric acid for proper digestion of protein, and, as shown in the study by Hennings, incompletely digested proteins may become a major source of irritation in rheumatoid conditions. We have to take care of digestion and assimilation in dealing with rheumatism and arthritis.

In the *Journal of Rheumatism and Arthritis* in 1983 a restricted diet was proposed for those with arthritis, eliminating or limiting intake of milk products, wheat products, red meat and caffeine drinks (such as coffee, tea and many commercial soft drinks). This is similar to the diet restrictions I have been using in my sanitarium work for nearly 50 years with excellent results. Wheat and milk products make up 54% of the average American diet. This is far too much, and any food that is taken in excess can be a problem in arthritic conditions.

I feel that the average diet in the industrialized nations of the

West, together with high-stress working and living conditions, strongly promote the general acidic conditions in the body that invite rheumatic disorders.

We find there are so many contributing causes and aggravating condtions to rheumatism and arthritis that it is evident that any permanent solution will take the form of a broad program of dietary and lifestyle changes. It is rare (if not impossible) to find a single cure for any disease with multiple causes.

There are many things to consider in correcting a rheumatoid condition or osteoporosis. There are no panaceas, no "silver bullets" that will stop these things with a single injection, pill or even health supplement. I feel the only reasonable approach to taking care of arthritis and other rheumatoid conditions is a program designed to take care of all chemical deficiencies and raise the health level of the whole body, so the body can take care of the condition its own way. I have had wonderful success with this program, and I believe you will too.

Contents

1

Let's Look For Causes

When we deal with rheumatism, arthritis and osteoporosis, we are more or less dealing in the same chemical realm of each one of these problems. All of these conditions come from the same chemical shortages in the body. We have to look at the causes of these troubles, because our work is one where we remove the cause, if at all possible, no matter how long it takes.

Rheumatism is the "family" of all acute, chronic and degenerative conditions that involve soreness and stiffness of muscles, pain in joints and related structures. It includes all types of arthritis.

Arthritis may be defined as joint inflammation associated with such widely varied conditions as infection, rheumatic fever, colitis, accidents, nerve and metabolic disturbances, glandular imbalances, kidney problems, dietary imbalances (such as too much meat in the diet) and psoriasis.

The basis for rheumatism and all the conditions it includes is chemical imbalance in the body, leading to a local or general acidic condition. I am including osteoporosis, increased porosity of the bone structure, because it, too, is related to the same type of chemical imbalance that can bring on rheumatic conditions. Osteoporosis may be associated with diminished estrogen, calcium deficiency and malabsorption, vitamin D deficiency, muscle wasting, lack of exercise and high intake of meat.

One of these days, doctors are going to study the conditions of older people with these diseases and find out that if proper treatment had been given 20 years ago, they wouldn't have these ailments today. Onset of arthritic symptoms may be sudden, but the body chemistry must have been "ripe" or they wouldn't have happened. This takes a long time.

These days, our country is going calcium crazy, and I believe many problems will be encountered because of it. Everyone is taking calcium supplements instead of getting it from eating calcium-rich foods. But, our bodies don't respond to the chemical calcium as they do to the bio-organic calcium in foods, which is taken in with other minerals, vitamins and enzymes. If calcium intake is not balanced with the proper intake of bio-organic sodium (again, as found in foods), spurs and unwanted calcium deposits may develop. Vitamin D, exercise and the proper glandular balance are necessary before calcium can be assimilated properly. Otherwise, we will get calcium out of solution, causing troubles in the body.

There has been quite a mixup in what most people have been taught about sodium. There is chemical sodium, such as in table salt, which may be considered a drug, and there is bio-organic sodium, as we find in foods. We need the bio-organic sodium to neutralize body acids, balancing the calcium, and it must come through out foods, not as table salt sprinkled on foods or already contained in foods as an additive supplied by the manufacturer.

My method of approaching the treatment of rheumatism, arthritis and osteoporosis is to use food and lifestyle changes as medicine. You must understand this idea before you can be well. You can use drugs to take away symptoms temporarily, but only foods can change your body to get rid of the cause of the problem. New tissue can be developed best with proper nutritional means.

Now, in taking care of these cases, we have to recognize that we have to compensate for what has been done in past years by the patient. I think one of the greatest problems of diagnosing or taking an analysis of a person, is to go back and see what kind of a life that person has led. Then we can begin to see what the accumulated effects are over a period of years.

No osteoporosis came on over night. No slipped disc came on over night. There is no rheumatism that begins to develop in the body that came by just having a cup of coffee or by having a donut or having some junk foods once in your life. It is an accumulated effect, and we have to recognize that, just as the Cancer Society says, it takes 20 years to develop cancer. Arthritis can be triggered by trauma, but there is usually a developing arthritic condition already existing. When an accident jars the joints and bones, it only hastens the bringing out of symptoms from a rheumatoid condition that has been lying latent or is just in the beginning stage.

Of course, I always ask, "Where was the doctor in the beginning?" It was in the person's lifestyle. It was in the person's habits. It was in the person's manner of living. It is found in his marriage. It is found in his job. It is found in his environment.

So, let us go back and check these things out and see how we develop them, and then we can begin to see how we are going to compensate for them. Then we probably will be able to live a life that is going to go just opposite to what we have been doing.

Sometimes we have to learn how to stop a habit that is breaking down the tissue structure before we can get well. It is very important to take on a new life, a new direction, a new path, when we find ourselves in these troubles.

I have talked and written about preventing diseases for many years, but sometimes it seems I don't get through well enough to my patients. For instance, with myself, I try to get as much as I can out of my body. It is one of energy, it is one of effort, and it is one of seriousness; it is one of achievement and accomplishment. And, of course, I use these faculties to the limit, not always realizing that when I overuse my analytical ability or my critical ability and my seriousness and sincerity, that I can overdo it.

Sometimes I think diseases come to tell us that it is time to reckon with the problem. But it is usually late in life when these problems come on. Then sometimes it too late, as it can be in cancer. It is very difficult to always go with the start of a problem and to correct it at the very beginning, especially in this day and age of living in the fast lane.

Technology is upon us in full swing, and as a result, we live a life of comfort, in the main, which, in the long run, takes its toll. Because the person who does what he feels is the easiest to do may not be the healthful person he wishes to be.

Of course, I am referring here to the amount of exercise we take every day, the amount of sunshine we have, the amount of resistance we put into life. I have heard many people say the only thing they want is something like love, success, achievement, so forth. The very thing they are striving for could be achieved if they had a different attitude, more positive and less negative.

Most people fight their diseases, and that very fighting makes the disease worse. Some people say they will try a certain treatment, but they try it with half a feeling it may help, and yet it may not. They must put every effort, interest and enthusiasm into the treatment before they will get well.

Sometimes we have to do twice as much for ourselves in order to get well, to break up the effects of some of the habits that have held us back in the past. Most people want to do just enough to get by, and this may not be enough to take care of the problem that has developed.

The first thing we must realize, though, is that any time we have a symptom of any kind in the body, or any discharge, any pain, any development of a calcium growth, like a spur, osteoporosis, a kyphosis or a scoliosis, we need to realize it has been coming on for quite some time. In the beginning, it does not cause much trouble. If it did, it was usually only a flickering pain—"Oh, it doesn't bother me." So, we get up and out and keep on going.

There are probably more women with these troubles and problems than men, but here also, they have something to learn.

Arthritis Is A Symptom: It Is Not A Disease

There are 20 different kinds of arthritis these days. There are so many types that affect the bones, some just the joints. Sometimes the bones get soft and some of the joints get stiff. As a result, we have all kinds of bone and joint disorders. Let me give you a few definitions here so you can understand them better.

Arthritis. Inflammation of a joint, usually accompanied by pain, and, frequently, changes in structure. The word arthritis comes from the Greek terms *arthron* (joint) and *itis* (inflammation). Arthritis is defined as an inflammation of a joint. Symptoms are local tenderness and redness, with pain and swelling, and local increase in temperature. Arthritis may result from infection or trauma. The joint may become stiff, sometimes due to fibrous connective tissue, cartilage or bone joining the articulative surfaces or to spasms of the muscles surrounding the joint. Chronic or rheumatoid arthritis is one of the most common of crippling diseases. Gout is a form of arthritis triggered by the settlement of uric acid in the joints, particularly of the legs and feet.

Osteoarthritis. A chronic disease involving the joints, especially those bearing weight. Characterized by destruction of articular cartilage, overgrowth of bone with lipping and spur formation and impaired function. Osteoarthritis is the same as degenerative arthritis, degenerative joint disease or hypertrophic arthritis.

A degenerative joint disease far more common than rheumatoid arthritis, and usually less damaging, is osteoarthritis. It apparently results from a combination of aging, irritation of the joints, wear and abrasion.

Degenerative joint disease is a non-inflammatory, progressive disorder of movable joints, particularly weight-bearing joints. It is characterized pathologically by the deterioration of articular cartilage and by formation of new bone in the subchondrial areas and at the margins of the joint. The cartilage slowly degenerates, and as the bone ends become exposed, small bumps or spurs decrease the space of the joint cavity and restrict joint movement.

Unlike rheumatoid arthritis, osteoarthritis usually affects only the articular cartilage. The synovial membrane is rarely destroyed, and other tissues are unaffected.

Rheumatoid Arthritis. Form of arthritis with inflammation of the joints, stiffness, swelling, cartilaginous hypertrophy and pain.

Rheumatism. A general term for acute and chronic conditions characterized by soreness and stiffness of muscles, and pain in joints and associated structure. It includes arthritis (infections, rheumatoid, gouty); arthritis due to rheumatic fever or trauma; degenerative joint disease; neurogenic arthropathy, hydroarthritis; myositis; bursitis; fibromyositis; and many other conditions.

Osteoporosis. Increased porosity of bone. Osteoporosis is a bone disorder affecting the middle-aged and elderly—white women more than men of black or white ancestry. Between puberty and the middle years, the sex hormones maintain osseous tissue by stimulating the osteoblasts to form new bone. After menopause, however, women produce smaller amounts. As a result, the osteoblasts become less active and there is a decrease in bone mass. Osteoporosis affects the entire skeletal system, especially the spine, legs and feet. As the spine collapses and curves, the thorax drops and the ribs fall on the pelvic rim. This position leads to gastrointestinal distension and an overall decrease in muscle tone. "Dowager's hump" is due to osteoporois.

Among the factors implicated in bone loss is a decrease in estrogen, calcium deficiency and malabsorption, vitamin D deficiency, loss of muscle mass, inactivity and high protein diets.

Not only arthritis, but also rheumatism and osteoporosis are almost always effects of some other cause in the body. It is important that we not only treat the effects, but more so to discover the causes.

I want to bring out in the very beginning of this book that all three of these conditions—rheumatism, arthritis and osteoporosis—are considered in the chemical classification. In fact, I strongly believe that every disease stems from a chemical lack in the body. Gout often comes on after years of excess use of alcohol and heavy protein meals. Drinking alcohol breaks down the kidneys, which then can't process uric acid as well. The uric acid (from protein) gets in the blood and settles in the joints. The way to get rid of gout is to stop drinking, cut down protein, get on a good exercise program and start a balanced nutritional program. We have to restore sodium in the affected joints. Whenever we have hardened joints, a lack of limberness, we find out then we are lacking sodium.

There is an extreme amount of acidity in all of the diseases that bring on these conditions. This usually comes from overwork, from living a tired life, not having enough time for ourselves, not having the proper hobbies to balance the daily routine and prevent overdoing in any one direction, even if it is in doing the right thing. We can even do the right thing too much without proper understanding.

Oftentimes, people don't get enough sunshine. Some have too much sunshine, and they don't balance their lives either. Problems can develop from the type of clothes we wear by not allowing proper circulation to the body, by not allowing proper circulation in the breast area; by wearing garters, belts, ties, so forth. We can wear the wrong kind of clothes.

We should perspire more than we do, three times a week at the very least. Some people don't exercise their bodies enough to get them warm. They live in a cold body constantly.

If a person would feel his knees, he will find out his knees are usually colder than any other part of the legs. The joints don't always have the same amount of circulation in them that the rest of the body does, particularly the muscle structure, unless a certain amount of exercise is taken every day. We must exercise. We will discuss that as we go along, especially in Chapter 4.

While I urge you to perspire at least three times a week, at the least, I don't want you to overdo it. A person who is constantly sweating is throwing off too much sodium from his body.

Therefore, he must have sodium drinks and sodium foods to put the sodium back into his body.

I had a patient one time who was one of the highest ranking basketball players in his league. He told me that he lost as much as 12 pounds by sweating in one night of play. Until he came to see me, he was compensating for this loss of sodium in his body with lots of juices, sweet water drinks, cola drinks and other types of commercial drinks that are probably high in sodium—but with the wrong kind, and they are very acid producing.

He was advised to take salt tablets, made out of regular table salt. But after he came to see me, I put him on foods high in natural sodium. This is the way we should be replacing the sodium salts that are lost in perspiration. Within a short time, this procedure corrected a lot of his problem.

While on the subject of sweating, let me comment on what some of my female patients have told me about this problem when they are going through menopause. Some of them have had to get up two or three times a night to change their nightgowns because they have been sweating so much. This excessive sweating is carrying off the sodium salts, and that leaves a calcium disturbance in their bodies. The calcium is coming to the joints and causing a distortion of the spine, in many instances, along with hunchback and scoliosis and curvature. Most always, it's resulting from a lack of balance of sodium in the body. The lifestyle is usually the culprit, bringing on a burning up of the sodium, leaving an extreme acidity. So Mother Nature does her best with what she has to work with.

In order to assist in this process, I recommend ripe citrus fruit and all other fruit and vegetable juices. However, with this one very important qualification: *It must be fully ripe!* If it isn't, it will cause kidney trouble in the long run. Why? Because it stirs up body acids and puts too much strain on the kidneys, overworking what is often a weak kidney system.

The sun is our sodium star. It has a very vital task—to ripen fruit. Most citrus fruits are picked six weeks too early. So, instead of the high sodium content which it should have, it ends up with an excessive amount of green citric acid. This stirs up all the other acids in the body, overworking the entire elimination system, especially the kidneys. While we need sodium, we do not get it if fruit hasn't been properly matured by the sun. Sodium, in nature, is sweet to the taste. Only a truly ripe fruit, fully matured, is the right fruit to put into your body.

Sometimes people have developed such serious conditions over a long period of time that degeneration sets in to such an extent, a hip joint is broken down. That makes it usually an irreversible condition, demanding surgical intervention, often with a total hip or knee replacement.

Proper body chemistry is so important I am devoting Chapter 2 to this subject. I will treat it there in much more detail.

2

The Proper Body Chemistry

As mentioned in the previous chapter, when acids are produced in the body, they burn out the sodium. Sodium is stored most in the stomach wall. When it is not there, we lack the digestive juices to digest and assimilate our foods properly. Sodium is very high in the bowel wall also, which takes care of digestion as well as elimination. When assimilation and absorption are poor because of lack of sodium, then we cannot absorb enough of the food elements for our body or keep the proper electrolyte balance in our bowel. We cannot keep the proper balance of sodium and calcium throughout the whole body.

We must realize that calcium is a very hard material, and it can settle in knobs on the joints and spurs in between the vertebrae. And, of course, when it does, it is always from a lack of the proper sodium in that particular area.

The Need for Sodium

Sodium is found to be the second highest in joint material. Sodium is robbed from the body by improper living habits and not having enough of it in our diet. This produces acids that steal the body's sodium reserves from the stomach and joints. Then symptoms of discomfort finally arise in these joints and the stomach. No one ever has joint trouble without also having a lot of stomach trouble, as well as absorption and assimilation problems, bowel troubles and a lot of gas.

Bloating and a dry stool are common. All kinds of intestinal disturbances begin to develop. I am speaking now of the very *causes* of the trouble, and these are what must be taken care of first.

The Need for a New Lifestyle

In taking care of the sodium lack in the body, we first have to stop breaking down that poor overworked machine. We have to take up a new path in life. We have to be really serious enough about it and convicted enough within our conscience to realize we have done wrong, and that the only thing is to go back and compensate for doing the wrong things in the past.

To compensate, we have to do the right thing for awhile, and that doesn't mean doing just a little bit or whatever you feel you can do. It has to be done on a persistent basis. It has to be done with perseverance. You will find that as you stick to it, eventually these troublesome conditions will leave the same way they were built up and came upon you.

To describe some of these problems, I emphasize that your past environment has a lot to do with them. People with lower back disturbances, what they sometimes call a slipped disc, those who have kyphosis (angular curvature of the spine), osteoporosis or calcium out of solution, so to speak, because of lack of proper sodium balance, have developed these disturbances over a long period of years of not enough exercise.

According to Dr. Fred McDuffie, medical director of the Arthritis Foundation, there are significant differences in the ways the two most common forms of arthritis (rheumatoid and osteoarthritis) affect those suffering from these disabilities.

According to the Foundation researchers, the typical person with rheumatoid arthritis faces 23 "bed days" a year, plus a higher risk of unemployment and divorce than the national average.

People with this kind of arthritis also experience an average of 7 days a month or 84 days a year of restricted activities.

Persons with osteoarthritis, however, can generally expect fewer consequences than persons with rheumatoid arthritis, reports Dr. McDuffie.

Osteoarthritis affects the joints, but is not as serious a condition as rheumatoid arthritis, which is often crippling.

One study showed that a typical person with osteoarthritis must spend 14 "bed days" a year.

We have all built up a certain kind or type of body, possibly with weaknesses in the lower part of the back. Sometimes we have been overweight. Many times, if we have been overweight, we have a weak back. Then we start a dieting program and rob our bodies of the proper amount of calcium and sodium. Then this weakness in the back begins to get even more pronounced, even weaker. We discover that as we diet and get less calories, we can cheat ourselves out of the proper chemical elements that the body needs.

Diet Fads

Some people go through many diet fads, not realizing that those diets were not properly balanced when they went on them. There is always a new fad being promoted. I wonder why. Could it be perhaps because when people find out they don't work, the "authorities" have to come up with a new one?

Some people cut out meat entirely from their diet, then discover they do not have enough protein, which is very much needed to build good joint material.

On the other hand, just mentioning this, somebody is going to say, "Well, I have left out the meat; now I am going to eat meat again." You can go without meat, but you must know what the alternative protein foods are before you can possibly go without meat entirely. If you have been a meat-eating person all of your life, especially if you cut it out all at once and not gradually, your body will go through a lot of serious biological changes.

You may have to go through an elimination process, because the body is going to make some adjustments according to the new diet you have undertaken. That is why so many people feel very wonderful going on a fast. A reducing diet is bound to make you feel better, temporarily, that is. The joints will feel better. Acidity is eliminated for the time being. But unless we go on the proper maintenance and build-up diet afterwards, we can start accumulating more trouble for the future. Dieting is something that has to be carefully weighed, and many times should be taken up under proper supervision.

The Need for Calcium

A person who is constantly going on juices, for instance, should probably have a lot of bio-calcium foods, because most juices are high in sodium, but many of them are very low in calcium. If we don't have enough calcium, eventually the bone material can begin to break down, holes begin to form, and it gets into the realm of osteoporosis.

Osteoporosis consumes the bony material that makes up our joints and bones in the body, while calcium spurs can be a result of an addition of calcium to the bony structure. Calcium can lodge in any joint in the body.

The lower back is probably one of the places most susceptible to having this problem, because of our occupations, whether they involve a lack of exercise or too much exercise. Osteoporosis usually develops in the lower back.

Arthritis sufferers need to have a greater amount of sodium for the joints than the average person takes. They also have to have a plentiful amount of calcium. Many people have the erroneous idea that because calcium spurs have developed, and joints have these calcified knobs on them, that they have too much calcium in the body. They believe they cannot eat more calcium foods. This is not always the case. What they really need is to have enough sodium to balance the calcium, so it doesn't come out of solution and deposit in the joints.

Sodium gives us the chemical material to neutralize the body acids. It is also the element that is stored in the joints that softens any hard material that may settle in the body in the form of calcium. Sodium keeps the body limber, soft, pliable and active as far as the joints are concerned. Since sodium is stored in the joints, you can rest assured if there is joint trouble and you develop any stiffness or if calcium develops or if anything is going out of place after a lifting job or an occupational job that is throwing the back out, *you are lacking in sodium.*

Sodium is a very important element to have in the body. So, when I talk about sodium, pay particular attention to that. And I don't mean the common table salt, as mentioned before, but that element which comes naturally from our food.

In order to give you a little help in this regard, I am listing below the three categories of foods you need to consume to overcome the problems I have been discussing. I suggest you make up your own menus from this list and follow one of my cardinal rules: *Every day, have 6 vegetables, 2 fruits, 1 good starch and 1 good protein.* While I have emphasized the need for sodium in this chapter, let me urge you to zero in on *whey*, which is one of the foods highest in sodium content.

Potassium Foods

Almond nuts
Apricots
Artichokes
Bananas
Barley
Beans, lima
Beef
Beets
Beet greens
Blackberries
Blueberries
Broccoli
Brussels sprouts
Carrots
Cauliflower
Chayote
Cherries, wild black
Chervil
Chicken
Chicory
Chives
Coconuts
Corn
Cucumbers
Currants, black
Dandelion greens
Duck

Potassium Foods (Cont'd.)

Eggplant
Endive
Figs, black mission
Grapes
Halibut, smoked
Honey
Horseradish
Kale
Kohlrabi
Lamb
Lemons
Lentils
Lettuce, sea
Limes
Mangoes
Mushrooms
Mustard greens
Olives
Onions, white
Parsnips
Parsley
Peaches
Peanuts
Pecans
Potato, baked
Prunes
Radish, black
Radish, red
Raisins
Spinach
Turnips
Watercress
Zucchini

Sodium Foods

Butter, cow
Cheese, Swiss
Chinese cabbage
Leeks
Milk, cow
Milk, goat
Okra
Papaya
Pears
Pineapple
Pomegranate
Pumpkin
Raspberries
Rice, natural brown
Squash
Strawberries
Swiss chard
Veal joint broth
Watermelon
Whey

Calcium Foods

Asparagus
Banana
Beans, lima
Blueberries
Bread, whole wheat
Butter, cow
Buttermilk
Brussels sprouts
Carrots
Cauliflower
Cheese, cow, cottage
Cheese, goat, cottage
Cheese, roquefort
Cheese, Swiss
Chinese cabbage
Chives
Cream, cow
Cucumbers
Dandelion greens
Endive
Grapefruit, fresh
Honey
Kale
Kohlrabi
Leeks
Lemons
Lettuce, Romaine

Calcium Foods (Cont'd.)

Limes	Parsley	Swiss chard
Mangoes	Peaches	Turnips
Milk, cow	Peas, fresh	Turnip leaves
Milk, goat	Pecans	Watercress
Mustard greens	Persimmons	Watermelon
Oranges	Pineapple	Whey
Parsnips	Strawberries	

I also urge you to get my latest book, *Vibrant Health From Your Kitchen*. This is a complete course in nutrition for the lay person, resulting from over 50 years of my clinical experience, world-wide travels, and my very latest discoveries in this fascinating field. If you can't get it from your health food store, have them order it from me at the address in the front of this book. This book goes into very great detail on the important factors enabling you to recover and maintain good health that I have only been able to briefly consider here.

Another one of my books I consider an absolute must for everyone is *Tissue Cleansing Through Bowel Management*, which you can also get from your health food store or direct from me. This book shows you dramatically how to clean out that malfunctioning septic tank you have. You didn't know you have one? Well, you do (it's your bowel), and in most people, it is backing up and creating one horrible mess. Constipation is our national disease.

I have often said what you get out of the body is often more important than what you put into it. It is impossible to be really healthy until you have a clean bowel.

The first edition of my *Tissue Cleansing* book has sold over 80,000 copies, which gives some indication of how many people believe its subject matter is important to their health.

You will notice in the tabulations of the food lists that some of them have more than one chemical element, but quite often they have just the one indicated in the heading. But if you want to zero in on just one element, then perhaps you should double up more on that particular food.

In this chapter, for example, I have been stressing the great need for sodium. But that is only if you are in special need of it. For the average person, it is far better to strive for a *balanced* dietary regime.

For the benefit of those who may have a little difficulty in making up your own menus, you can get much help by referring to my book previously mentioned, *Vibrant Health From Your Kitchen*. It contains many menu suggestions covering the full spectrum of proper chemical elements for a well-balanced dietary program.

In the next chapter, I will discuss an important factor, the need for a satisfying occupation and its impact on your health.

3

The Occupation Problem

I would now like to take up a discussion of the occupational side of the health problem. Many people don't realize that their occupation can be the seat of many of their difficulties these days, especially if you hate your job.

One important element is where you neglect to get the amount of sunlight that should be coming to the body every day. These folks who are living away from sunlight, such as in offices all day, have an artificial light coming through the pupil, which is robbing the body of vitamin A. They are not keeping a proper balance so the joints can be limber, soft and pliable. They are the ones who are usually wearing glasses. When they do get outside they find in wearing glasses they are keeping the ultraviolet part of the light spectrum from entering the body through the pupil of the eye.

Most glasses (those that are true glass) screen out about 85% of the ultraviolet from the sunshine coming through them. Ultraviolet light is what we used to treat rickets and pronated ankles in children. Rickets is a sign of a lack of calcium. It is quite possible we may be producing some of that lack by the type of glasses we wear. I personally believe in plastic lenses. They allow in as much as 85% of the ultraviolet, which is just the opposite of the regular lens glass. This is one of the first suggestions I make—to change regular glass to plastic lenses.

Get Plenty of Sunshine

The next suggestion is to get outside as much as possible and spend as much of your time as you can in the sunshine. My Oregon and Washington friends tell me this is a little difficult in their states, for they say there are only two seasons: August and the rainy season! This may be an exaggeration, but those folks do have to put up with probably the most rain in the country. They also tell me the only people who can be happy there are those who have webbed feet! So, if you aren't a duck, stay away from damp, wet climates especially if you are prone to arthritis.

If you work in an office all day, you are under artificial light. In that kind of environment, the body cannot get the proper material to control the calcium in the body. So you must compensate by getting out in the daylight as much as you can. There are a full spectrum of fluorescent bulbs available on the market, so I suggest you confer with your supervisor to find out if he can have them installed. They are far superior to the ordinary bulbs.

You must not strive to get an extreme amount of sunshine, because, for certain types of people , it can be harmful if overdone. There is ultraviolet light all around in just a shaded outdoor setting when the sun is shining. It can be a reflection from buildings, hills, flowers, wherever you may be. This is something that doesn't take place in a dark office or when you wear glasses and live under artificial light all day long. It has been said that a 10-minute sunbath will give you all the vitamin D for your body to last 3 days.

I feel sorry for those people who work in a building that is eight stories high, or more, in one square block, such as in San Diego. It hasn't a single window in the whole place. Imagine people going into these buildings, working a full day at a typewriter or computer, using their eyes. They are producing acids in their body. (And, by the way, all work produces acids in the body.) If you work under pressure, under the influence of dissatisfaction, dissension, you are producing a lot of acids. Far more than you would if you love your job or were getting along fine with the boss or are happy in your environment, in your working conditions.

If you are so far behind in your work that it is disturbing you constantly and you feel you will never catch up, it is just another acid-producing condition that can surround you.

When people come out of this building in San Diego that I mentioned, they have to go home. They are interested in getting home as soon as possible. They are on the freeway fighting traffic. They have to stop and go; they have to be alert; they have to be overalert, actually, and they overuse their nervous system. If you get in the 55-mile-per-hour lane, most of the drivers are doing 65 and 70. So you have to watch every turn and every move of the person in the car near you, besides taking care of your own driving.

Not only that, but you are sitting in an automobile, usually, with closed windows. If there is any light to come to you, you are cheating yourself of the ultraviolet light that is being filtered through the glass in the car windows.

We are behind glass most of the day. We live in a glass house, so to speak. And I do believe this can be the beginning of a lot of our troubles.

The Sedentary Life

There are a lot of people who have to sit all day long at their jobs. I think sitting can be the cause of most of our lower back problems. We don't sit in the proper chairs, in the first place. Manufacturers make different chairs—straight-backed chairs, kitchen chairs, curved chairs, chairs that allow your feet to touch the floor and some that don't let your feet touch the floor. Some people are built with short legs and they don't fit the average chair. As a result, they sit in a strain all day long. This is always bothersome to the lower back. They are building up a weakness because of their occupation.

Now what do we do to compensate for this? We have to exercise every day. And we must exercise enough so that we don't have an additional problem added to any inherent weakness, now that we have taken on the beginning of our new life. This inherent weakness will show up sometime or other because of our acquired living habits throughout our life.

Consider that you always have your inherent weakness, the inherent shape you have built. Sometimes it can be quite abnormal, with all the bulges and extra weight. Even being underweight can sometimes be an inherent possibility that we have to work with and consider. We have to have a certain amount of exercise to compensate for these occupations and how we live.

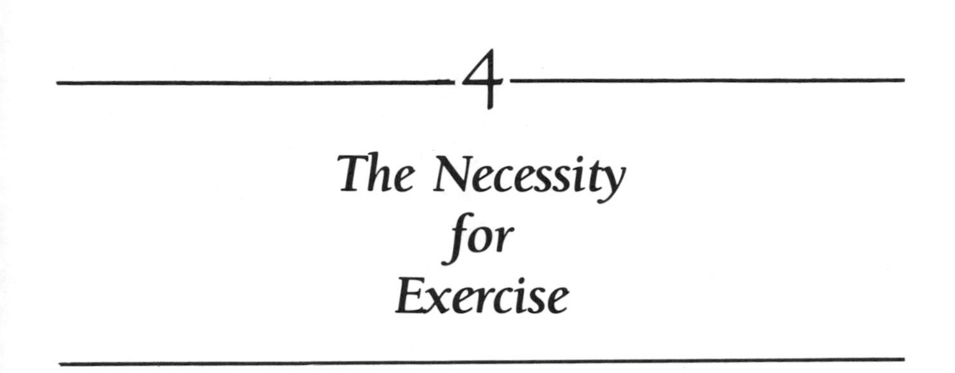

4 The Necessity for Exercise

My first thought regarding exercise is to make sure we don't do it in the over-abundance bracket. We should be able to exercise a little every day to keep the body limber eough, flexible enough, so that we can keep active on any job we have to do. It is not a matter of becoming a Mr. or Miss America. It is a matter of having a good limber, pliable body throughout. And that is why I feel that in exercising we should extend ourselves and our muscles. We must extend our joints to such a degree that they are kept quite pliable, limber and movable.

My first recommendation is to follow the Figure 8 exercises described in detail. While food is important, when taken in proper quantities, qualities and balance, you don't cure your infirmities through food alone. Exercise is equally important. Those that I call Figure 8 exercises take care of all bodily joints so spurs can't form and no individual calcium deposits can settle in any one place of those joints.

All Figure 8 exercises follow a circle pattern. The reason calcium spurs develop sometimes is because we don't use circular motion enough. When we walk or jog, our joints move back and forth, not around and around as they should. Figure 8s are *corrective exercises* and should be done every day. Diet and exercise work together in *natural harmony*. Exercise without a proper diet is not wise.

The Figure 8 exercise system is the best system I know for the joints. They are carefully thought out and put together so you can get the greatest amount of good from them. You can also bring these exercises onto a bouncer if you want to. Figure 8 exercises are the best way I know to keep the joints limber and flexible. They move the blood and lymph in the joint areas. They have been used by dancers for many years, and they will work just as well for you. Most people find them fun to do, especially to music. Repeat each exercise 3 to 6 times.

FIGURE 8 EXERCISE FOR THE KNEE JOINTS

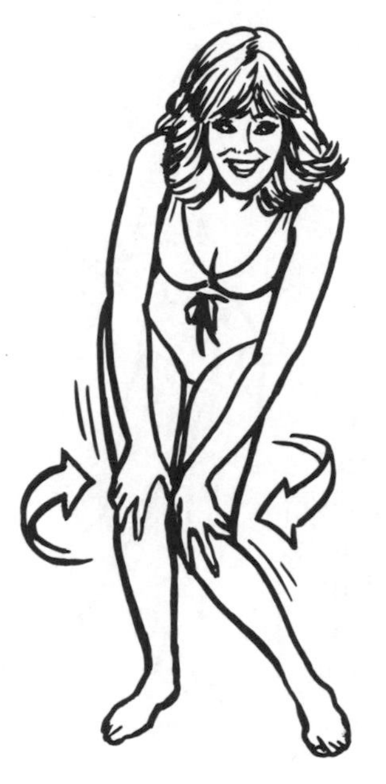

Move the knee joints in a circular motion by bending knees slightly, moving in circles or "figure 8" motion in each direction. Work up to 10 times each day (placing the hands on knees for balance is helpful). This knee exercise uses all sides of the joints not normally used, and keeps them pliable, limber and supple.

HIP JOINTS, FIGURE 8 EXERCISE

Stand with feet 6 to 8 inches apart and visualize a figure 8 on the floor. Stand in the center of the "8" and move hips and buttocks in circular or figure 8 motion in each direction. Work up to 6 to 8 times each direction. Make the figure 8 motion as large as possible to left and right sides. It is almost like the hula dance movement.

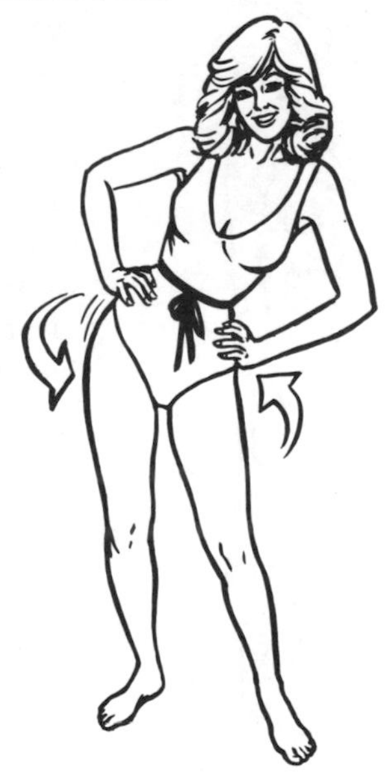

SHOULDER JOINTS, FIGURE 8 EXERCISE

Visualize a figure 8 around your shoulders. Move shoulders in figure 8 motion each direction. Lead with right and then left shoulders. Work up to 10 times each direction.

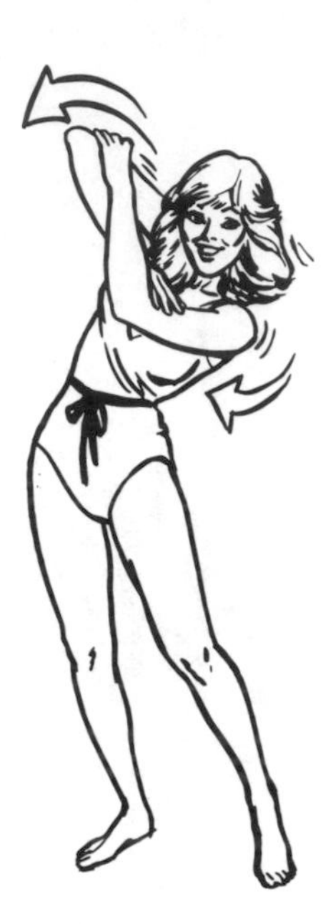

SPECIAL 8

A good figure 8 exercise follows one used by Fred Astaire, the well-known dancer and actor. He moves from side to side, lifting one shoulder and rising on his toes, then he follows the shoulder around in a circle. As he drops the other shoulder, he raises the arms and makes another figure 8. This exercise stretches the spine, coming up to compress the organs on the other side. Repeat 3 to 6 times on each side.

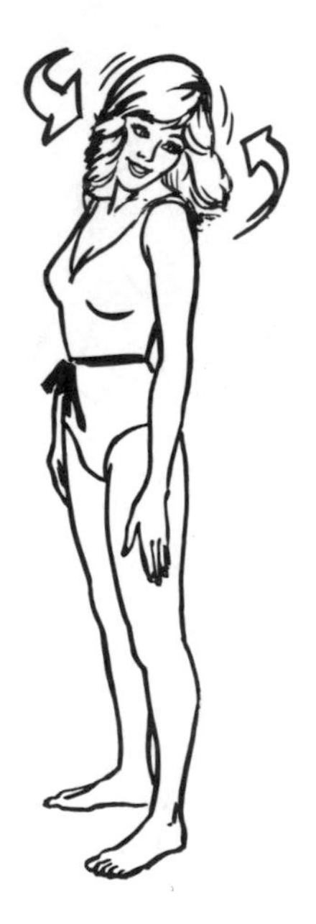

NECK, FIGURE 8 EXERCISES

This exercise is similar to the ancient Persian dance "neck loops." Look straight ahead. Do not look to either side. Slide the head straight over to the right side in the figure 8 or circular motion. The neck is over the shoulders, so to speak, a different movement than used in everyday movements and in different directions. Keep eyes and head looking straight ahead.

Exercising the Extremities

Now we go to some other exercises that may help. I believe the fingers should be exercised well. This can be done by squeezing a rubber ball. Moving your feet in time with music, let your body sway—what was the old saying, "swing and sway with Sammy Kaye—" do this while flexing your fingers and hands with arms above the head, down at your sides, extended like airplane wings, out in front of your body, behind your back. Work those fingers in time with the music in quick, flexing movements to exercise all the little muscles. You can continue the hand exercises in some of the other bouncer exercises, if you choose.

Toes and Ankles

Lift up on your toes, swing your heels in and out (toward one another, away from one another). Then bring the heels down and swing the knees (held closely parallel) in circles to the left and to the right.

Knees

As you do these exercises, bend and straighten the knees, flex those knees, not removing your feet from the bouncer or the floor if you don't have a bouncer, and jog gently from the knees only.

For those who may be overweight, I suggest you get one of my latest books, *Slender Me Naturally*. It contains many more exercises that you will find helpful. But for those of you who aren't overweight, if you will do those listed above, you will find they will help your joints a great deal. As I mentioned before, proper diet without exercise is not wise. The two go together.

By doing all of these exercises, I know you will get excellent results for the hands, fingers, knees, legs and feet. They will exercise your joints admirably.

Arthritis and rheumatic conditions usually start in the extremities. They can result from poor circulation. Many people have cold hands and feet, and in these cases, the circulation is poor in the extremity joints. These people do not have enough blood getting into the extremities to repair, rebuild, regenerate and recuperate. This can be accomplished wonderfully through exercise.

When we want a new body in place of the old, we can't consider just hot packs, massage or exercise alone. We cannot even consider just good thinking, important as that is. We cannot be all spirit. We cannot just pray. We've got to get off our knees and do something about our health problems. Our prayers have to be in the form of work. What does the Bible say? Faith without works is dead. Our bodies were meant to be used. As the old saying goes, if you don't use it, you lose the use of it.

Now this can also be taken care of partially through the use of certain supplements in our body, which I will describe later on. And especially taking care of the thyroid gland when we have a low metabolism. But there are other things to be done besides taking supplements that we accomplish through our exercises.

Brisk Walking

A brisk walk is something that most anyone can do. Of course, if you have severe arthritis and you are in bed with it, you have to do your exercises while in bed. You have to move that body even though you are bedfast. When you do not move it, then arthritis can settle even more in your body, in the joints rather than any other part.

This reminds me of the current Lipton tea television ad. Two men are working out on exercycles. One of them says to the other, "I'm all worn out. I can't do any more." Whereupon his partner says, "I have just the thing for you." He brings out a big pitcher full of ice cold Lipton tea and says, "This is just what you need. It's brisk." After taking a drink, the pooped out partner says, "Boy, this is great, I feel terrific." His friend replies, "Fine, let's do some more exercise." Which brings on the response, "Well, I don't feel that terrific—just good."

What I want to happen to you is not to feel just good, but terrific! And you can, if you will follow my program outlined here.

The Ethel Lesher Story

One of the most amazing recoveries I have ever seen in all of my clinical experience is the Ethel Lesher story. As my latest book, *Vibrant Health From Your Kitchen*, relates, Ethel Lesher was nearly disabled with arthritis at the age of 76. After taking up a food regimen and program I gave her, she left the arthritis behind and started playing with a dance band she organized. She has appeared on the Johnny Carson show and played the piano on one of our shipboard cruises, at the age of 98! Ethel's story should be a great inspiration to those who feel that chronic diseases automatically come with aging.

"I took a trip in 1961," she said, "and when I returned, I was weak and my knees were swollen. I had been healthy most of my life, but I became rundown from doing too much. Besides taking care of my ranch, I was active in five different organizations. So I went to my doctor, and he told me I had arthritis. He said we all get it as we grow older. We just have to live with it.

"That kind of stirred me up. I didn't want to live with it. So I tried different things to get rid of it, but the arthritis just got worse."

Some years before, I had given a lecture in Redding, California, on "The Path to Right Living," and Ethel had attended that lecture. At the time, she was having such difficulty she remembered my lecture and decided to come to my Ranch in Escondido, California, to see if there was anything she could do for her arthritis.

The program I gave Ethel included vitamin B-12, jacuzzi baths, cold water Kneipp baths, barefoot grass walks and a food regimen that included high sodium foods such as whey, celery and okra to bring the calcium deposits in her joints back into solution in her body.

After two years of sticking to my program, the arthritis left. "I thought I would never play the piano again," Ethel told me, "but gradually I was able to get back to it."

She began playing with a band which included a drummer, tenor saxophone and banjo—for senior citizen groups. One day, she received a phone call from the local veterans' hall asking if she and her band would be willing to play at a Saturday night dance. Their music was so well enjoyed that they continued playing there on Saturday nights for three years. The crowd that came to dance tripled in that time.

During that time, Johnny Carson heard about Ethel's band and asked her to appear on his Tonight Show. What a wonderful thing that was for a woman in her 90s, once almost crippled from arthritis!

When she joined our shipboard cruise a few years ago, Ethel not only played the piano for us, but showed everyone she was still a good dancer. She danced with the ship's social director and had a great time on the cruise.

Ethel watches her diet carefully and follows what she learned at my Ranch, eating a variety of fresh vegetables and fruits, with eggs, poultry and fish as her main proteins. She keeps her bowels regular, is physically active and has many friends.

Recently, Ethel Lesher celebrated her 100th birthday with a gathering of friends and relatives, and this is what she had to say when she was asked to speak to the group.

"Dear relatives and friends, I love you all. I'm so happy to be here, and you have all been so nice to me. I just want you to know that my nutritional doctor, Dr. Bernard Jensen, couldn't be here. If it wasn't for him, I wouldn't have lived as long as I have.

"Thanks to Dr. Jensen, there isn't an ache or pain in my body that prevents me from enjoying everything, everywhere I go. I wish everyone could be as free of aches and pains as I am today.

"When I first went to Dr. Jensen's Ranch, my knee was swollen, my finger joints were bumpy and I could hardly use my hands.

"He told me, 'You've got to live a different life.' Dr. Jensen told me what to cut out of my diet and what should be in it. He gave me a program to follow. He said that he couldn't do a thing for me unless I made up my mind to follow a different path of living. I didn't want to be a cripple, so I made up my mind to do what he said. I had determination.

"For two years, I walked the straightest line you ever saw, until every ache and pain left me. I had no more. From that day to this one, I have felt wonderful. Today is my 100th birthday. If I had to ride a horse, I could do it.

"I want you to realize, too, what music has done for me and what I think it can do for everyone. Music is not only for the home, but for the heart and for sharing with others. When you're sharing music with others, you're also enjoying it yourself. It's doing a lot for you. It's very seldom that a day goes by when I don't play the piano just a little. I don't forget playing with the dance band. I just enjoy it very much.

"I'll leave you with this thought. There's a lot of good in knowing about nutrition. But knowing won't do you any good if you don't determine to follow what you know and change your way of living. I feel so sorry when I see people crippled up with arthritis, and I believe many of them wouldn't have it if they lived right and determined to change their ways. I believe if I can do it, most others can, too."

Isn't this a wonderful story? Here is another example of a remedy with full tissue recovery, leaving a chronic disease and all its symptoms behind. The greatest thing I can say is that I agree with Ethel. If people are willing and determined to change to a right way of living, almost any health condition can be changed.

I have seen pain leave people where they have been told to go home, forget it, just attribute their difficulties to getting old. This is just not true, as Ethel Lesher's story proves. It results from a lack of the proper chemical elements in the body and from the proper lifestyle that they have neglected during their life.

This reminds me of the story of an elderly lady who went to her physician complaining about severe arthritis pain in her right knee. After giving her a thorough examination, the doctor said he could find nothing organically wrong with her, that it was just old age coming on and she would have to learn to live with it.

Whereupon she told him, "Doctor, I've lived 65 years. My left knee is just as old as the right, and it doesn't have any pain."

Exercising can be extended in many different ways. Swimming is very good. But I feel that a brisk walk can be done by virtually everyone, even an elderly person. It was Presidents Hoover and Truman who were taught by their doctors how to walk and to do brisk walking, and to do this with arms swinging, which helps the entire body, the circulation especially. It is something we should consider and do constantly, every day.

Three times a week, we should exercise enough to bring up a sweat. This helps the elimination process through the skin—which is the largest eliminating vehicle in the body. The skin must be taken care of as well by exercise.

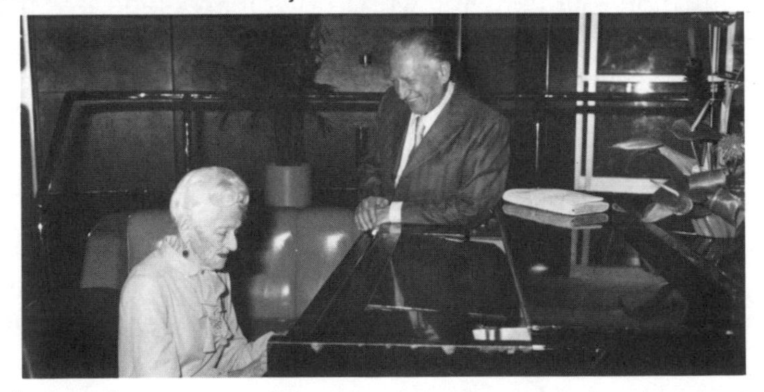

Ethel Lesher, at age 96, gives Dr. Jensen a demonstration of her piano style during a shipboard cruise.

Skin Brushing

The best thing you can do for your skin is to brush it with a vegetable bristle brush. The brush exercises the little muscular pores that the body has wherever there is hair on the skin. As we brush those little pores, we develop the muscular structure so it can throw off toxic material through the skin area. I have never found a person who has perfect skin activity.

Poor skin function comes from wearing clothing, in most cases, especially when we wear nylon clothes. They prevent the absorption of the toxic material from perspiration.

The toxic material that comes from the skin daily equals the amount excreted through the bowel daily.

Taking a regular bath every day also is important to develop the tone of the pores. The skin has to be kept active the same as the bowel or any other eliminative organs. In taking your bath after your morning exercises, a shower, for instance, take a warm one, but end up with cool water passing over your body. This is done to close the pores, but it is also a form of exercise.

I believe that the Kneipp water baths are some of the finest that a person can get acquainted with. We can go still further and use shiatsu in our treatments, to make sure we break up all of the mental toxic-spotted tension points that may have developed in our body through our job, our marriage problems, strain or stress, etc. Then, of course, there are chiropractic treatments. Without the proper nerve supply in the body, we cannot rebuild and regenerate the tissues. But, correction of chemical imbalance must go along with it. Without proper dieting, no other single therapy is going to do the job.

Osteopathy is very fine, but *all* forms of treatments merely offer temporary relief. Correcting a problem has to be done through proper dieting, to stop breaking down the chemical loss in the body which occurs through improper lifestyle.

Most of us burn out the chemical elements in our bodies through an imbalanced mental activity in our daily lives. It is this imbalance that we have to correct by getting back to a proper chemical balance. This is most important.

So, follow the proper diet, the few ideas given here, as we go along. You can follow it without too much trouble.

The Mini-Trampoline

I would like to bring out here that the mini-trampoline is a wonderful tool to work the muscles, to get a little bit of perspiration started. It almost acts as a substitute for jogging. Those people who have a lot of arthritis in their bodies do not believe in jogging, and neither do I, just as I do not believe in a lot of movement of the joints when arthritis has settled in them.

You first have to start by taking care of the proper diet, dissolve some of the hard material that is in the joints through imbalanced chemistry, through proper dieting and proper chemical supplements. Then, finally, use a little bit of exercise, and you will find this will help the body greatly. The exercise should come when your body is in a chemical state that will start dissolving the calcium as you begin to loosen up through your exercise program. All three conditions (rheumatism, arthritis and osteoporosis), should always start with the dieting program first. As you begin to dissolve the deposits, you will get a better bowel action, a better elimination process.

Exercise is needed by everyone including those with arthritis—even osteoarthritis or rheumatoid arthritis. You should consult with your doctor about the exercises you want to do, to make sure you can do them safely. People with arthritis can usually do many types of exercise—if they do them slowly, gently and gracefully. Studies have shown that a certain amount of exercise is necessary to prevent excess calcium loss from the spine and other major bones, so despite initial discomfort, exercise can help bring wonderful changes in many cases of arthritis.

Lymph is moved into the joint spaces by exercise, particularly by circular-type movements. Lymph fluid is high in sodium, and when this fluid circulates in the joints as it should, calcium spurs and deposits will not develop. It is only when the joints become stiff and blocked that calcium imbalance develops, and deposits begin to build up. Proper diet is one way we work toward chemical balance in the body, and this helps to dissolve hard calcium. But we also need exercise, together with diet. Exercise and diet together work much more thoroughly in restoring an acidic body to normal and in removing calcium deposits from the joints.

In all of my travels throughout the world looking for the oldest people, I never found an old man who had a stiff body or who was bent over. I discovered that the longest-lived old men, and sometimes women, worked out in their fields, bending over, lifting, pulling, and doing hard work that kept their bodies limber. Most of us, in our technological age that we now live in, have specialized jobs where we don't balance our bodies like some of the elderly people do.

In traveling all over the world, I have probably visited more old people than anyone else I know. And I can tell you they don't have stiff bodies when they get physically old. This idea that stiffness goes with age, or that you are supposed to have arthritis as you get older, is not true. I have taken care of many people who have had arthritis and gotten over it. Exercise and correct diet were the keys to their recovery.

Rebounder exercises to music introduce a level and type of physical activity that most people can take. Three to five minutes on the rebounder is equal to a mile of jogging, and every muscle in the body is exercised *without subjecting the joints or bony structures to the sudden impact shock that takes place when running or jumping on a hard surface.*

Many years ago, after visiting an osteopath in Hawaii who had a full-sized trampoline in his backyard, I designed a mini-trampoline for use by my patients long before the bouncers and rebounders so popular today were available.

We had a policeman at the Ranch who was on an early retirement due to an intervertebral disk problem that affected his back and neck, giving him a great deal of pain. I started him out on the bouncer with very easy exercises, gentle movements. He could do them without any problem, although he felt a little pain the day after his exercises. With my encouragement, he persisted and gradually increased the time and vigor of his exercises more and more. In a few weeks, his problem was corrected. This is what got me started on the rebounder exercises and showing my patients how to do them.

Rebounder exercises are actually tension-relaxation exercises. Our bodies tense as our feet land on the flexible cover of the rebounder and relax as we go into the air. This is what does our bodies so much good. The routine on the bouncer is a very important part of my own exercise regimen, and I enjoy this very much, always bouncing to music.

We Must Be Kind To Our Joints

The great thing about these rebounder exercises is that they are easy on the material that makes up the joints, and this is very important. Many exercises are harsh and jolting to the joints, compressing and stretching the soft inner material too much.

We must be kind to our joints because they say you are as young as your joints, and if they have been abused or if the diet is out of balance, they can become stiff, inflamed and painful.

The soft inner material of the joints is extremely sensitive to the acid/alkaline balance of the blood. If the blood is too acid, calcium spurs may develop. We must realize that incorrect diet and overexercise are harmful to the joint material.

Our exercises should never be so strenuous or overdone that more acids are produced than our diet and elimination channels can take care of, or our joints will be affected. We should never, in our lifetime, go beyond what our bodies can handle or we will find there are consequences to our health. For this reason, diet and exercise should be well harmonized.

I usually start out with Lawrence Welk's *Memories*, then go to the organ version of *The Happy Wanderer,* and last, something I like with a faster beat than the other two. You can substitute other music, but make sure the rhythm and tempo increase through the three songs or pieces you choose. It is best to record these three tunes on tape to run consecutively, so you can just turn on your tape recorder in the morning and get right into it. The time is about ten minutes for three pieces of music. You can increase the length of the music if you wish by adding other tunes later, after you are used to the ten-minute starting program given here. I recommend the albums or tapes of *Hooked On Swing* or *Hooked On Classics*.

There are more than one set of exercises. Learn one—do it, then learn another and do this one. Then you can do 2, 3, 4, 5 combinations. Your daily exercise routine shouldn't take longer than half an hour.

Bouncer

The main purpose of these exercises is to move the lymph and carry off the broken-down products of fat metabolism. These movements firm the buttocks, help reduce the waist and strengthen the legs. Be inventive. Make up some of your own dance movements as you go along. The object is to use as many muscles as possible and to move as many of the joints as possible.

Turn on your music!

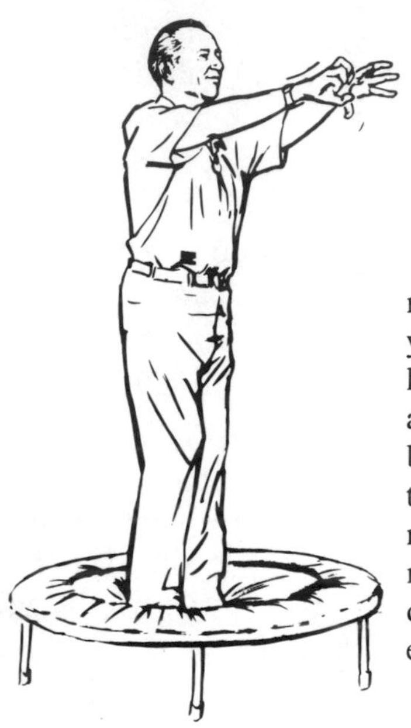

HANDS

Moving the feet in time with the music, let your body sway while flexing your fingers and hands with arms above head, down at your sides, extended like airplane wings, out in front of your body, behind your back. Work those fingers in time with the music in quick, flexing movements to exercise all the little muscles. You can continue the hand exercises in some of the other bouncer exercises, if you choose.

TOES AND ANKLES

Lift up on your toes, swing your heels in and out (toward one another, away from one another). Then bring the heels down and swing the knees (held closely parallel) in circles to the left and to the right.

KNEES

As you do these exercises, bend and straighten the knees, flex those knees, not removing your feet from the bouncer but "jogging" gently from the knees only.

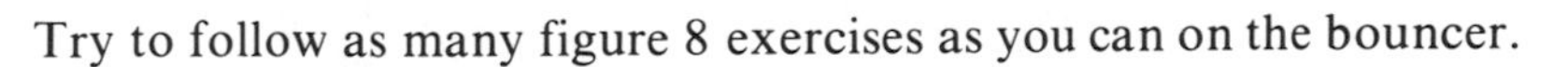
Try to follow as many figure 8 exercises as you can on the bouncer.

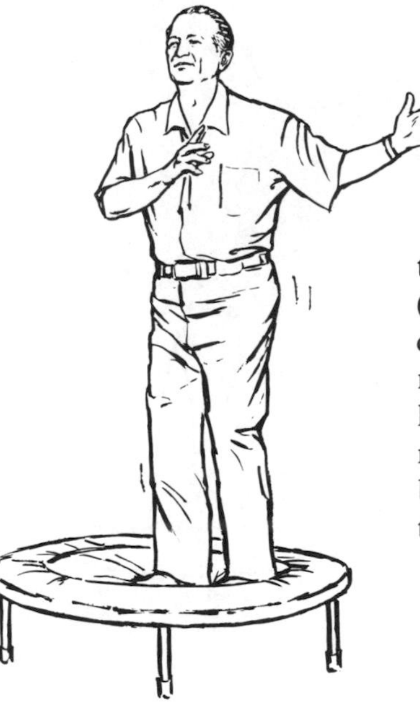

HULA HIPS

Move those hips in circular motion, then side to side, then front to back (thrusting the pelvis forward, then drawing it back), several times each motion. Move the arms in graceful hula-like motions, keeping the hands parallel, rolling the shoulders to work the upper body. Bring in the knee movements and the hand flexes.

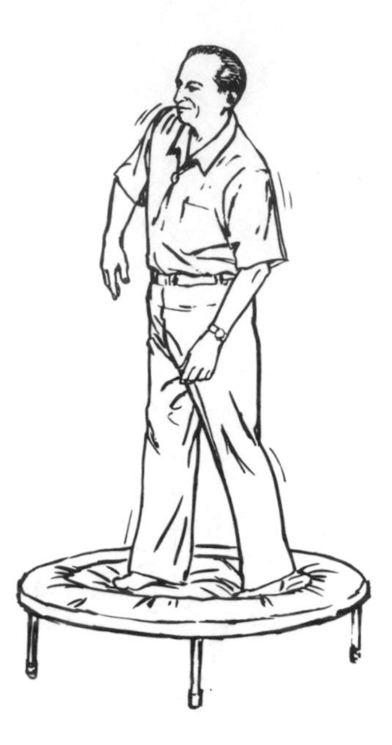

SHOULDER ROLLS

Drop hands to sides and rotate the shoulders alternately, left shoulder, then right shoulder, repeat, etc.; rotate in forward circles several times, then reverse circles, then do both shoulders at the same time, forward and reverse. Keep the legs going, the knees flexing, the hips swaying as you do this.

SWIMMING

Make swimming motions with the arms while keeping the feet, knees and hips moving—move the body continuously.

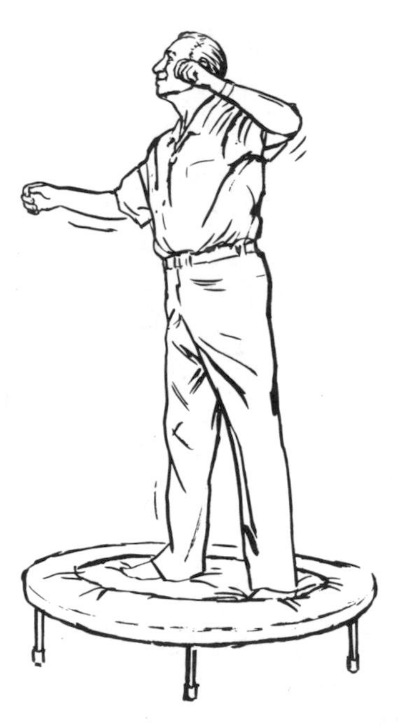

TWIST AND BEND

Twist the body from side to side several times, bend the body slightly forward, slightly backward several times.

NECK ROLLS

Move the neck from side to side, front to back, like a Persian dancer. Rotate hips in circles, the knees, the arms.

EYES (Not shown)

Hold the head still and make wide circles in the air in front of you, first with one hand, then the other, following your hands with the eyes. Repeat, closing the fist and making circles with one finger, following the finger with the eyes as you trace large circles clockwise then counterclockwise, first with one hand, then the other. Repeat 6 times each way. Then turn on the bouncer until you are squarely facing one wall. Again, holding the neck and head still, look from the upper right corner of the wall you are facing to the lower left corner, MOVING THE EYES ONLY. Shift the eyes to the upper left corner, then to the lower right. Repeat 6 times. Then shift the eyes to the right and do the same thing.

FIGURE 8 EXERCISES

The bouncer is a fine place to do the figure 8 exercises, and you may want to use them as part of your bouncer routine instead of doing them separately.

As the music shifts to the second tune, repeat the preceding exercises to the faster beat without lifting your feet from the bouncer. Do shoulder and arm movements like Fred Astaire or Ginger Rogers when they danced, especially the figure 8s with the arms and shoulders.

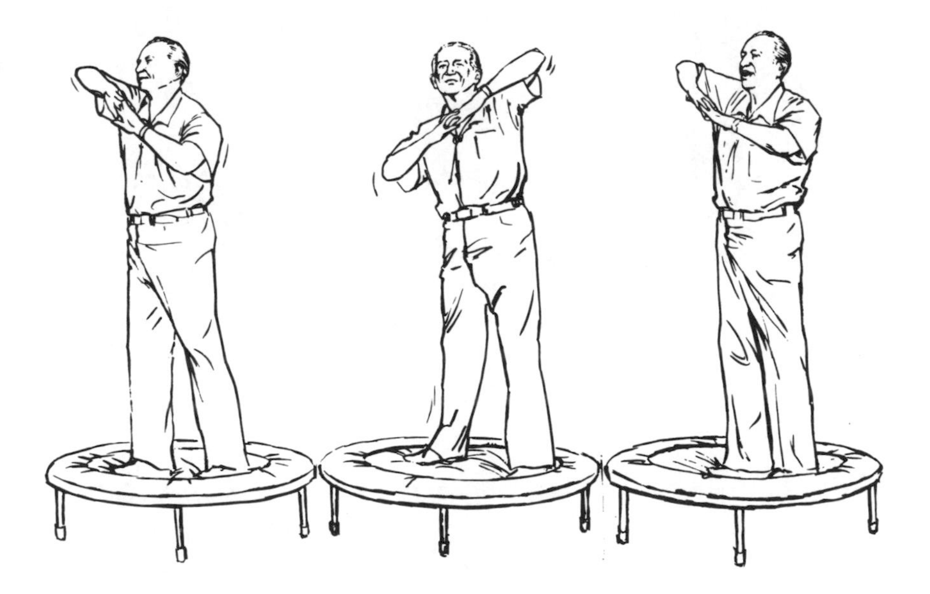

Do the hula hands, hula arms again. Move those feet! Repeat all hand and arm movements in the first four exercises. Move the hands in large circles in front of your face, one hand at a time, keeping your eyes on your hands without moving the neck. Do clockwise and counterclockwise circles. Keep moving in time to the music.

By the time the third and fastest piece of music comes on, you'll be warmed up enough to increase your activity level. When you increase the amount of time you spend on the rebounder, use it on this faster beat since you don't need any more of the warmups. Later, when you are able to use your rebounder to its limit, the more active exercise will increase your basal metabolism and continue to burn up more calories all day.

Repeat the movements as described in the first part of this section, but ***vary the foot movements.***

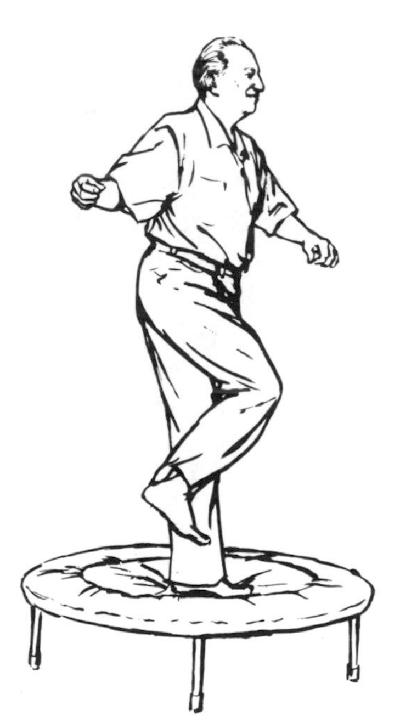

KNEE CROSSOVER

Cross the right knee over the left and bring it back. Repeat, crossing the left knee over the right 6 times each, alternating.

PIGEON-PENGUIN (Not shown)

Point toes together, heels apart, bounce. Then bring heels together, toes apart, bounce. Keep it up 6 times, alternating.

CHARLESTON (Not shown)

Do the Charleston, with small steps, so you can keep balanced; do 6 times.

KICKS →

Kick forward, one foot, then the other. When you kick, reach down toward the toes of the kicking foot with one hand, 6 times.

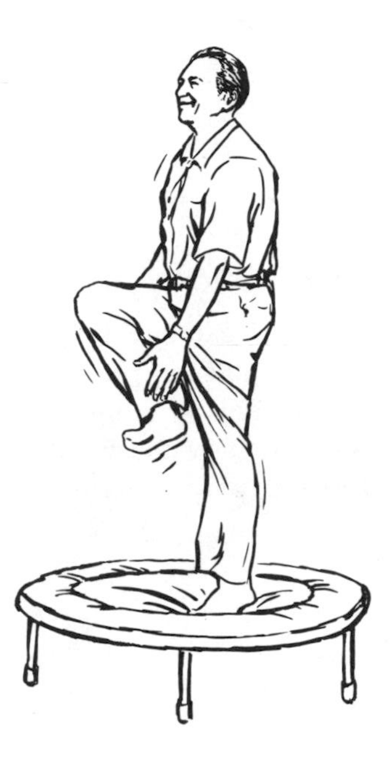

BELLYUP-BELLY DOWN
(Not shown)

As you bounce up, bring both hands to the lower-left abdomen and lift it a little as you go up and down, about 6 times. Then move the hands to the lower-right abdomen and repeat. Again, holding up the middle of the abdomen. You can do this with high jumps if you are comfortable in the process.

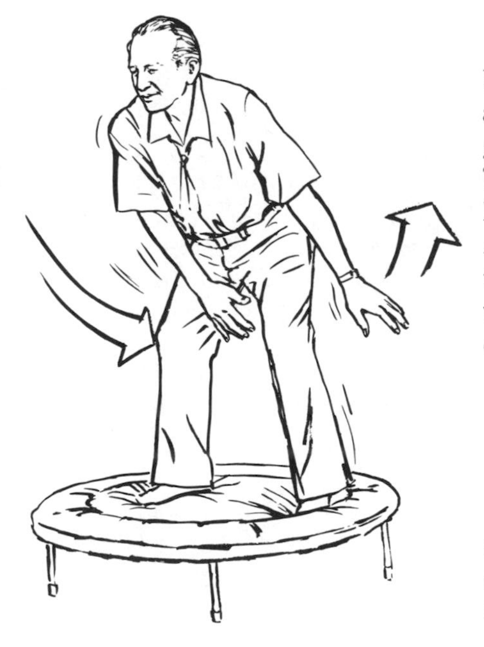

← *ARM CIRCLES*

Bend at waist, hands together, swing arms from side to side while bouncing on the mini-trampoline.

JUMP KICKS (GOOSE STEP)

This exercise helps to develop your balance. Kick your legs forward as if running. This is a bouncing exercise kicking legs forward.

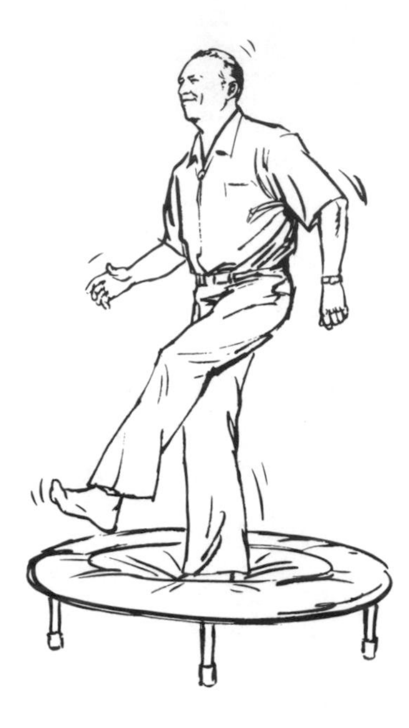

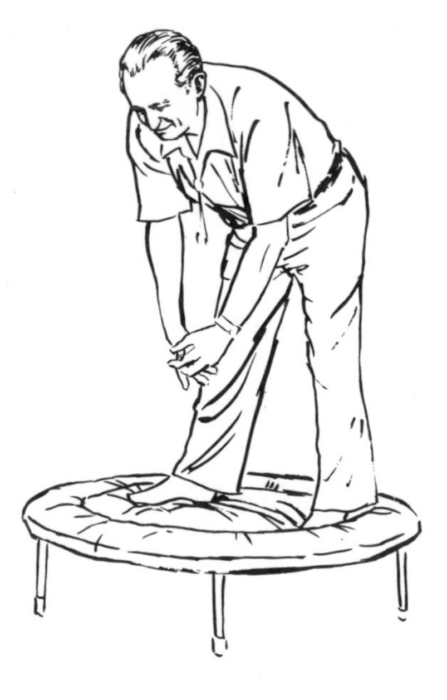

THE ELEPHANT

Clasp the hands, bend slightly forward and, with the feet apart, swing both arms to the left, then to the right, just as an elephant swings its trunk from side to side. The movement should be a graceful but energetic arms-and-shoulder stretch to one side then the other.

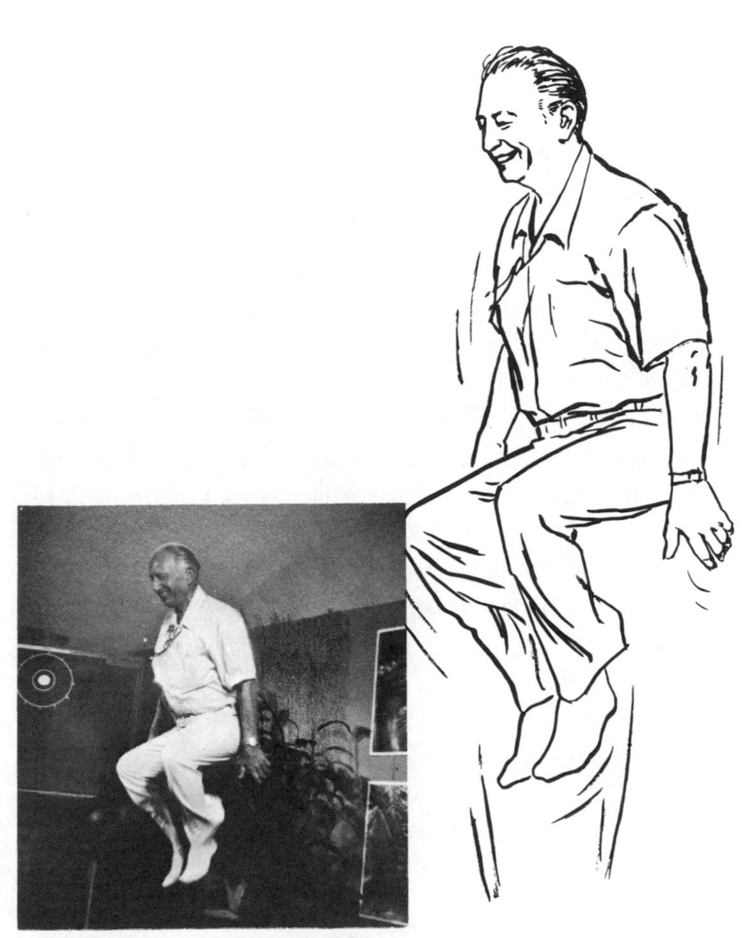

Dr. Jensen enjoying part of his daily bouncer routine.

After you get used to these, dream up your own bouncer routine with any movements you like, including dance movements. When you are by yourself, be creative, let fantasies go into action. Just be aware of the flexibility and limited foot space of the bouncer. I can't begin to tell you all the nice things you can do on a bouncer, but I want to encourage you to make up some of your own exercises and have a good time with your bouncer!

After you get used to these, dream up your own bouncer routines with any movements you like, including dance movements. When you are by yourself, be creative, let fantasies go into action. Just be aware of the flexibility and limited foot space of the bouncer. I can't begin to tell you all the nice things you can do on a bouncer, but I want to encourage you to make up some of your own exercises and have a good time.

Exercise is the most important process in taking care of lymphatic congestion. The lymphatic system consists of the spleen, thymus, appendix, tonsils, lymph vessels, nodes and fluid. The fluid moves by muscle contraction during movement. Lymph fluid must be kept moving to carry off the acids that irritate the joints.

If you are thirsty after exercising, add a crushed watercress tablet to your water or take an organic potassium tablet, so your body will not hold liquid. *This is especially important for those lymphatic types who retain water so easily.* Also you may wish to take vitamin B-6 which has been recommended by health researchers to help keep the water down in the body. *Do not take more than 500 mg per day without talking to your doctor.*

There are plastic suits you can buy to increase perspiration while you exercise and afterward. Ask your doctor about this, since for some, this may not be a safe procedure. *Perspiration is good for elimination of subcutaneous toxic material, but too much liquid loss can upset the chemical balance of the body.*

Perspiration helps to rid the body of acids, so that is another reason why it is necessary to exercise.

As far as water treatments are concerned, I believe that the hot and cold foot baths are the very finest. Put your feet in hot water for one minute, then in cold water for one-half minute. Do this five times, and do it twice a day.

If your hands are giving you a lot of trouble, put them in hot epsom salt water in a basin and leave them in the hot water and exercise them. By exercising the hands or the body in cold air, where the blood is not in the joints, you will find, many times, that it will irritate the joints. But, if you exercise them when they are in hot water, there will be a relaxation and expansion within these joints so the new blood can get in there and start doing a good job.

It will also do a good job if you will eat right and live right, along with it. And make sure that the elimination processes are well taken care of.

The Slant Board

One final thought on the subject of exercising that I consider most important—the slant board. The only people who should *not* use it are those who have heart trouble, high blood pressure, internal bleeding or those who are pregnant. It is sometimes well to have supervision in using the board. An extreme slant board or backswing are pieces of equipment I do not recommend without having proper instruction or supervision.

You can make your own slant board and put it on a chair which is about 18 inches high. I believe this should be a daily program if you can possibly get up and down on the board, especially if you have any arthritic condition at all. There isn't anything that will stretch and separate the intervertebral disks like the slanting board. If you can lie on the board—it doesn't have to be the extreme—you can start out with only 6 inches high at the foot end. If you use your own board, be sure to put a 2 or 3 inch wide strap across one end. (The commercial products have such a strap.) You will find that by keeping your feet under the strap, it will create a slight stretch on the vertebrae which hold the cartilage between them. As you stretch each day, even twice a day, you will find that that little stretching will help to rebuild that cartilage between the vertebrae.

If you are eating the proper foods and promoting the circulation by exercise, it is quite possible you will develop a new growth of the tissue between the vertebrae. As you grow older, it is more difficult, but you will find you are never too young or too old to begin this program.

If you make your own board, as I said before, start from only 6 inches of foot height, then gradually go to 18 inches, which is normal chair height. This is high enough if done every day. If you can do it twice a day, with the exercises I am giving you below, they will be a great help to you. I suggest you use a rubber ball also in a circular motion on the abdomen 25 times, then patting on the abdomen and then pulling the abdomen down to the shoulders 10 to 15 times. After exercising, lie on the board for 10 minutes to relax. This will start helping the tone of your internal organs in the lower abdomen.

Suggested Slant Board Exercises

Follow instructions carefully. You can feel relaxed, refreshed and invigorated quickly by stimulating circulation to all parts of the body. Do not try to do too much at first. Take on more exercises gradually. Do not attempt exercises that might endanger physical condition. If in doubt, have a physical checkup.

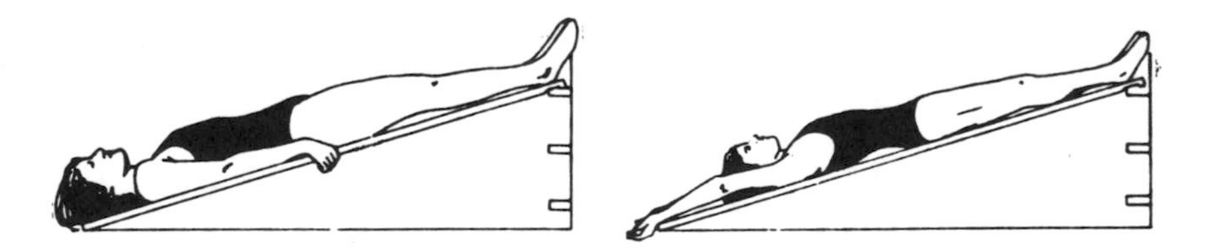

1. Lie full length, allowing gravity to help the abdominal organs into their position. Lie on board at least 10 minutes.

2. While lying flat on back, stretch the abdomen by putting arms above head. Bring arms above head 10-15 times. This stretches the abdominal muscles and pulls the abdomen down toward the shoulders.

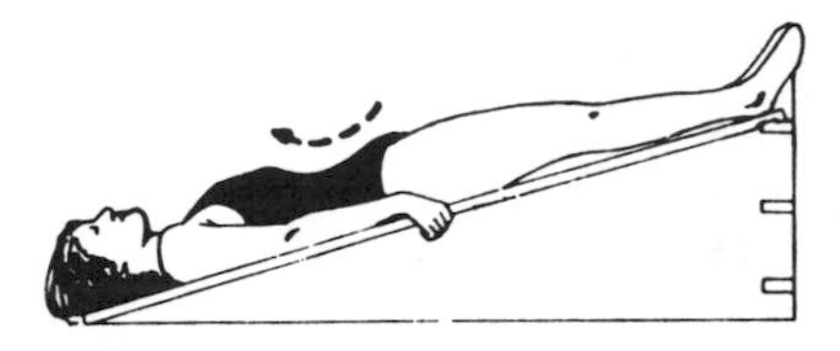

3. Bring abdominal organs toward shoulders while holding breath. Move the organs back and forth by drawing them upward, contracting abdominal muscles, then allowing them to go back to a relaxed position. Do this 10-15 times.

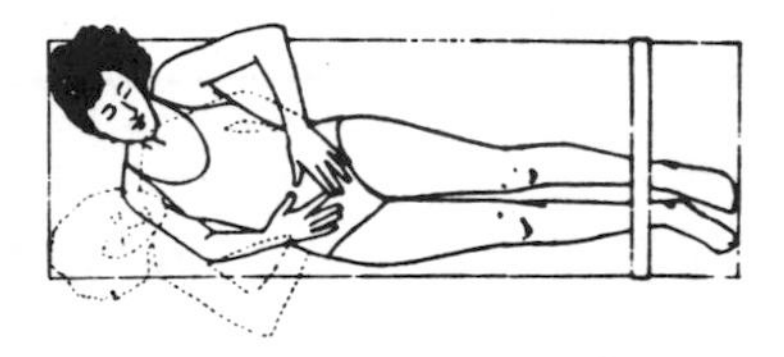

4. Pat abdomen vigorously with open hands. Lean to one side then to the other, patting the stretched side. Pat 10-15 times on each side. Bring the body to a sitting position, using the abdominal muscle. Return to lying position. Do this 3-4 times, if possible. Do only if doctor orders.

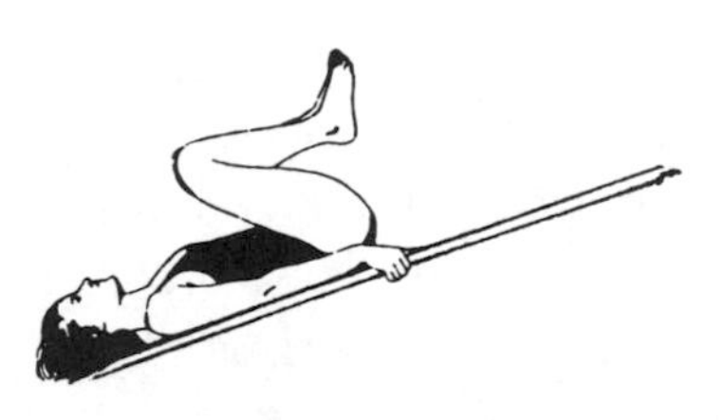

5. Bend knees and legs at hips. While in this position: (a) turn head from side to side 5 or 6 times; (b) lift head slightly and rotate in circles 3 or 4 times.

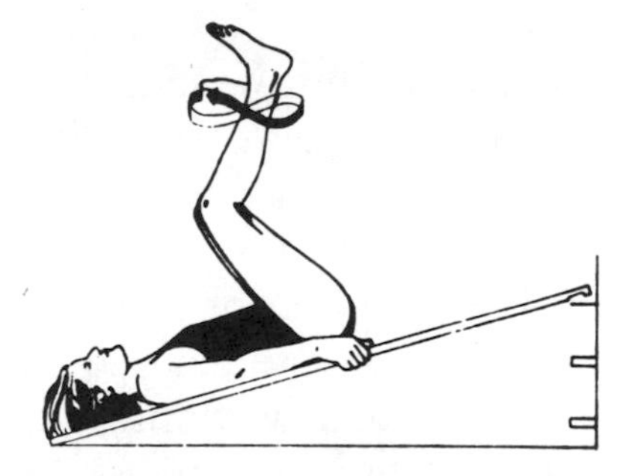

6. Lift legs to vertical position, rotate outward in circles 8 or 10 times. Increase to 25 times after a week or two of exercising.

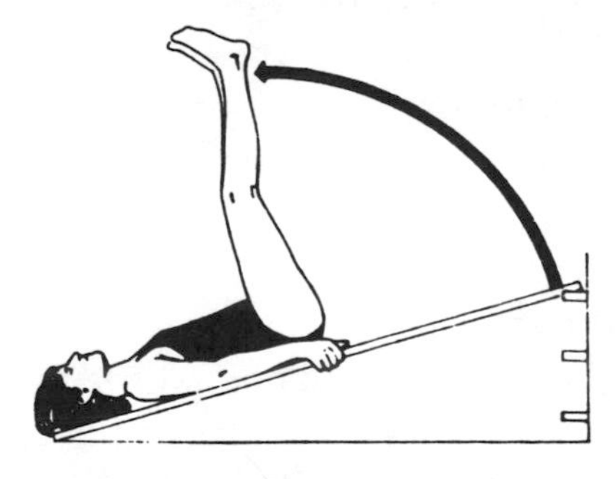

7. Bring legs straight up to a vertical position and lower them to the board slowly. Repeat 3 or 4 times.

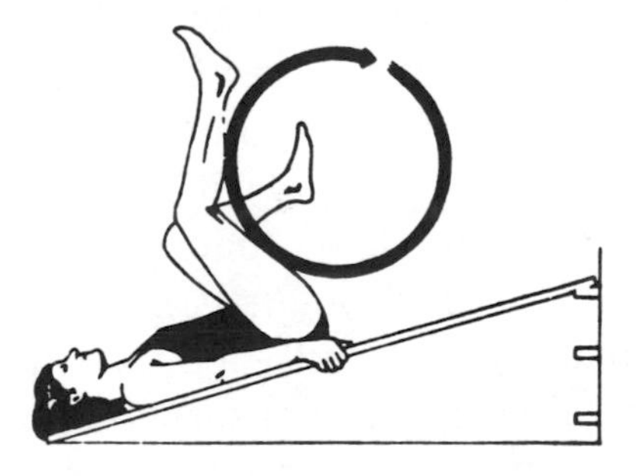

8. Bicycle legs in air 15 to 25 times.

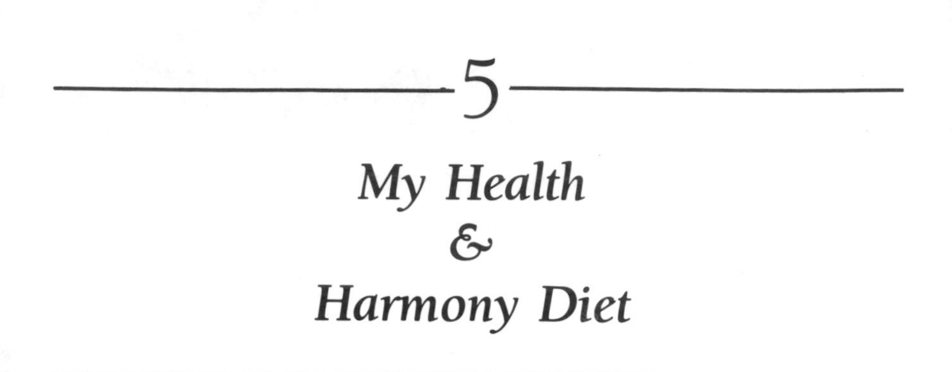

5 My Health & Harmony Diet

The next thing we must think about and take care of is the diet program. I suggest you follow my Health and Harmony Food Regimen which has been explained in several of my other books. I will summarize this program here for you. Let me suggest again that you get a copy of my latest, *Vibrant Health From Your Kitchen*. It is an up-to-date version, so those following my past program will find a lot of new things added, such as new food laws and especially the law of excess. I feel you should follow this program implicitly as a maintenance eating program.

If you want to go on the Eleven-Day Elimination Diet, all right. If you want to go on juices three or four days, either vegetable or fruit, all right, but essentially get on to this healthy way of eating program.

The main thing now in the diet is eliminating heavy amounts of table salt from foods. The *natural* sodium salt that you should have in your diet will come primarily from whey, as well as the supplements that I will talk about in another chapter. I suggest you refer to the food chart mentioned earlier.

First of all, you must cut out all junk foods. Try not to have too much wheat, milk or sugar. All three of these cut down on your digestion, your absorption and assimilation. They eventually produce an intestinal tract problem that can be found with all arthritic, rheumatic and osteoporotic problems.

All diseases have a catarrhal settlement with them. All diseases come with an excessive amount of acidity. With toxic joints, they produce a lot of catarrhal discharges in the body. Careful study of my Health and Harmony Food Regimen and my latest book will help you to take care of arthritis, rheumatism and osteoporosis.

Here is a new suggestion in the specialized food I suggest you eat. Black mission figs are high in sodium. Raw goat milk is high in sodium. You can also use kefir with the black mission figs. These can be used in place of a meal any time, or can be used in between meals in case you get hungry. They make a high sodium combination.

Strawberries and their juice, especially when they are ripe, are extremely high in sodium and can help the body. They can be used in addition to the diet in the form of dessert and special treats. They should, of course, be eaten without sugar. Practically all fresh fruit is high in sodium.

Sodium comes to these fruits because of the sodium star—the sun. The sun ripens them and creates the sodium development in the fruit and juice. However, if they are picked too early, the sodium hasn't matured. Immature fruit can cause a lot of irritation in arthritic and rheumatic conditions.

The greatest thing I can tell you is to cut out *all citrus* fruits, in spite of the fact that they are one of the highest foods in sodium. If citrus is picked too early, the sodium hasn't matured from the sun, and you are eating a green citrus acid. So eat only that citrus that is *fully ripe*.

As I mentioned before, I live in a citrus belt, and I can tell you that most citrus is picked four to six weeks too early. So you are not getting the sodium balance from that type of fruit when you take it into the body.

In addition, it is very irritating to the kidneys to put this immature citric acid into the body. It stirs up the acids and adds to the acids you already have in the body and forces the kidneys to take it out. If you have an inherent kidney weakness, and those organs have been overworked by your acquired past lifestyle, you will find you are adding trouble to the kidneys by having unripe citrus fruit.

If you can get organic grown, fully matured oranges or grapefruit, occasionally it is perfectly all right to eat them. Note that I said *occasionally.* But you should not have them every day. Variety is a food law.

There are several other fruits high in sodium that are listed in the previously presented food list. I do not approve of rhubarb, cranberries or plums in the diet, especially if you have arthritis. All three are very high in oxalic acid, and especially when you cook them, it becomes even more pronounced. We cannot have too much cooked spinach or Swiss chard either. They are also very high in oxalic acid. So having these greens occasionally in the diet—and raw—isn't going to hurt. But there again, they must be taken *occasionally.*

Okra and celery are two of the highest vegetable sodium foods. Many times, fruits stir up the body acids a little too much. So if we can sometimes lean to the vegetable kingdom and its sodium foods, you will find you will not stir up the body acids, and your rheumatic condition will not be aggravated by taking these fruit acids.

Vegetables carry off the acids; fruits stir them up. In arthritic cases, fruits give a lot of trouble, so you should go more to the vegetable juices, such as carrot, celery and parsley. This makes a fine combination.

I must tell you that alcoholic beverages of any kind aggravate arthritic conditions. It is best to avoid them altogether.

In the next chapter, I will cover the controversial subject of supplements—do we need them or not?

6

Do We Need Supplements?

A few statistics. 90 million patients visited a chiropractor last year. 53% of those were for low back problems.

2 billion people will be treated for low back pains in the next years (totaling from 1976).

20 million Americans suffer from gallstones.

Dr. Maynard Murray (M.D.), says: "You and I, fellow Americans, hold the dubious distinction of being among the sickest of populations in modern society. We are the best fed, chemically starved, people in the world."

He adds: "Despite our wonder drugs, steroids, sanitation standards and general medical wizardry, the United States has one of the highest infection rates per capita of any society, perhaps even higher than India, a nation that we are trying to help with our medical know-how, sanitation practices and pharmaceutical advances.

"There is no excuse for 97% of Americans having some kind of chronic dental disease. That's a terrible statistic; it's damn near everybody."

The above are quotations from Dr. Murray's revolutionary book, *Sea Energy Agriculture*. In it, he tells the fascinating story of how he traveled the world seeking the solution to our disastrous agricultural policies that have almost completely destroyed our soil.

He tells us that our cropping practices, plus the drainage of soil nutritients into the oceans have made our food grown in America, and the world too, for that matter, virtually valueless.

His solution was to take the purest ocean water he could find anywhere in the world (Baja California), dehydrate it, and use the resulting salts for fertilizer, both in soil and hydroponics. He has achieved almost unbelievable results, proven by dramatic pictures in his book.

Dr. Murray says that all of the body's chemicals are in perfectly balanced suspension in the ocean, so why not take them from that source and rejuvenate our soil? His is the first promising light on the agricultural horizon, and may well, in time, bring about a radical improvement in world agriculture.

Our ancestors a couple of centuries ago had no need for doctors, hospitals, drugs and all the other paraphernalia of modern medicine. They knew nothing about supplements, vitamins, minerals, etc. Whenever they had need of medical assistance, they called on an age-old wisdom of using herbs, Mother Nature's natural remedies.

While I don't decry the marvels of modern medicine and surgery, I feel we have gone overboard and need to get back to a simpler way of life. We have literally gone drug crazy and vitamin crazy. Much of this has been implemented by high pressure advertising.

Look at the TV ad that shows a person holding his hands about six inches from either side of his head saying, "I had a headache this big, but I took such-and-such pain reliever, and now my headache's gone." This is typical of all drug advertising. It makes us expect *instant relief*—not cure. It *suppresses* the symptoms and leaves the underlying cause still there—to be suppressed all over again and again and again whenever the symptom reincarnates, as it will. That relief is only temporary, and the treatment makes us a drug addict for the rest of our life. Unless. . .

We drastically alter our lifestyle, as I have constantly advocated in this and all of my other books, so we eliminate the cause and not forever treat the symptoms. For once we eliminate the cause, there will be no more symptoms.

Many health-minded people have become thoroughly disillusioned with the false promises of drugs and have switched to vitamins and minerals. And especially they are looking to so-called "organic" products. They don't realize that the laws of most states say that manufacturers can call their products "organic" if they contain only 1% to 2%—the rest being synthetically produced.

Now I want to discuss the supplements we should or should not add to our diet in order to be well, in order to balance our bodies chemically. The first thing to consider is calcium, which must be added in most cases, in spite of the fact you already have calcium in the body. There are very few man-made calcium supplements of which I approve. The calcium-magnesium balance is usually poor. One brand will be too high in calcium, too low in magnesium; another is too high in magnesium and too low in calcium. The electrolytic balance is not considered. Any time man tries to be king in nature, I have to doubt the kinds of things he has developed.

I feel that the bone meal calcium tablets are the best. Bone meal is a whole food. It is made of the joint material, and it is the joint material that we have to replace in the body. It is at the end of the joints that we consider a protomorphogen that will replace the joint material that is broken down in a rheumatic, arthritic or osteoporotic person.

When we have slipped disk problems, the disks come out over the vertebral edges, because, as we get older, we find the vertebrae get closer to one another. This is because of gravity. The exercises referred to in another chapter will help to separate the vertebrae so that a great amount of building process will take place in the joint material. So I suggest you review that chapter now.

Bone Meal and Whey

I believe that taking four bone meal calcium tablets two times a day is a necessity for most people. But I feel that with the sodium foods that I suggested you should now take another sodium food, which I approve of very much. It is one called Whex, a dried goat whey. It can be purchased from the Mt. Capra Cheese Company, 279 S.W. 9th Street, Chehalis, Washington 98532. A testing laboratory report for this product is included here indicating how high this food is in potassium and sodium. By the way, potassium is also an alkalinizer in the body. Most people who have kidney, heart or bowel problems, are in need of potassium, which this food concentrate will supply.

Goat whey, in this concentrated form, should be taken as one tablespoon in a cup of warm water, with a tablespoon of lecithin granules. Take this twice a day. Make this a ritual and follow through for a period of time. It has taken at least five years to bring on rheumatism, arthritis or osteoporosis in the body, and it will take you at the very least a year to catch up with a lot of careful, right living and lifestyle. You are trying now to compensate for what you have done in the past. You are trying to speed this up by giving yourself the extra things you should have had all through the years.

Veal Joint Broth

One of the greatest foods that will help arthritis, rheumatism and osteoporosis is veal joint broth. Now this, you may say, is meat, but I might tell you that a real meat broth is high in uric acid. Meat contains the uric acid, which can be harmful in many cases of arthritis, rheumatism and osteoporosis and also in kidney problems. But there is no uric acid in veal joint broth. It is made strictly from the joint material, and it acts like a protomorphogen, which means we get life from life. And since we are using a

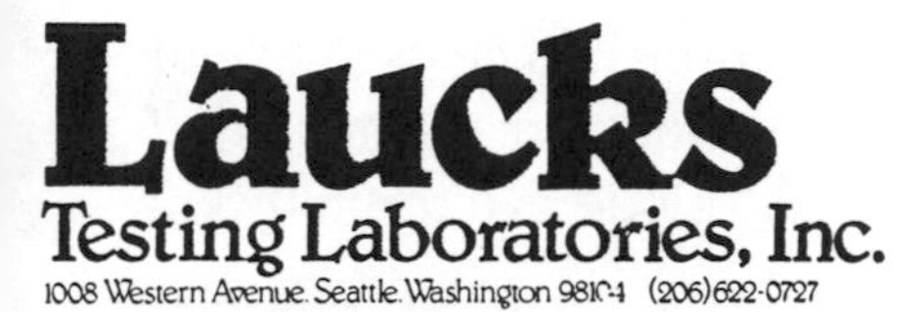

1008 Western Avenue. Seattle. Washington 98104 (206)622-0727

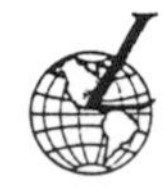

Certificate

Chemistry, Microbiology, and Technical Services

CLIENT Briar Hills Dairies
279 S.W. 9th
Chehalis, WA 98532

LABORATORY NO. 73419

DATE June 19, 1981

REPORT ON GOAT MILK WHEY

SAMPLE INDENTIFICATION Marked: 1) Whex Dehydrated Goat Milk Whey
Net. wt. 6 oz.

TESTS PERFORMED AND RESULTS.

Briar Hills Dairies has changed their name to Mt. Capra Cheese Co.

Ash, % 9.3

SEMI-QUANTITATIVE SPECTROGRAPHIC ANALYSIS
(on ash)

Potassium	41.%
Sodium	4.0
Phosphorus	3.1
Calcium	1.1
Magnesium	0.79
Silicon	0.58
Boron	0.012
Aluminum	0.037
Manganese	0.0043
Lead	0.015
Iron	0.068
Tin	Less/0.0031
Lithium	0.0043
Copper	0.0054
Titanium	0.0076
Silver	0.00035
Strontium	0.0054
Chromium	0.0054
Other elements	nil

Respectfully submitted,

J. M. Owens

JMO:ks

This is an analysis of a concentrated goat whey called Whex. I use this a lot with my patients.

material that is already organized by the animal, to be used by our body, our digestion doesn't have to sort it out, reassemble and digest the food and make it into what the blood can use. Thus, it will finally become our joints.

Doctors have been using protomorphogens for years. They use prostate for prostate; they use ovarian substances for ovarian troubles; they have been using thyroid substance for thyroid troubles. So now, we use joint material for joints. Like attracts like. And the God-given center in your body absorbs and takes the material it needs when you furnish it.

I want to emphasize this point: that when you furnish the body with the proper substance, it will take it up. But if you do not furnish it, the body cannot assemble it into the proper chemical combinations. It is necessary to realize that nature will cure, but she has to have the opportunity to do it. Your opportunity comes now in the food ideas I am giving you.

Free of Pain

I want to devote some time now to let you know about the remarkable work of John Marion Ellis, M.D., who has written a book titled *Free of Pain*. His findings are based on 20 years of clinical experience in treating ideopathic carpal tunnel syndrome. Doesn't that sound impressive! Translated, it simply means arthritic-type pains in the wrist.

These pains can become so severe that grown men sit on the edge of a bed at night in such agony that tears flow freely and they pound their fists on the wall in frustration. The usual treatment is an operation to reduce the nerve pressure. But Dr. Ellis has developed a simple method of treating thousands of patients with no surgery or drugs but only by use of a simple vitamin: B-6. He recounts many fantastic cures in his book.

Dr. Ellis is also a strong advocate of natural foods. This type of diet is the main element of preventive medicine, a principle he has always known and believed in. He is a strong advocate—just as I—of eating our vitamins in foods.

He says that among the B-6 rich foods that can be eaten uncooked are brewer's yeast, wheat germ, bananas, pecans and avocados. A banana has been found to be five times richer in vitamin B-6 than any other fruit.

Dr. Ellis also says, "It was an exhilarating feeling to know that I had discovered a cure for one of man's commonest problems, particuarly as the cure involved no drugs, no restriction of diet and no excessive expense. For a few pennies a day, a patient could be restored to health, with fingers that flexed painlessly and arms that moved easily.

"Thousands of my patients have been taking B-6 for many years, all without any ill effects. I felt confident that no possible side effects would occur, because B-6 is a water-soluble vitamin. Any excess above body needs is excreted in the urine within eight hours. Unlike fat-soluble vitamins such as A and D, vitamin B-6 cannot be stored in the liver."

It is so encouraging to know that there are pioneers in the orthodox medical profession who are beginning to realize that drugs are not the answer. Only foods can rebuild and repair body tissues.

Dr. Ellis makes quite an understatement when he says, "I had already discovered that the medical profession and the scientific community are solidly set in their beliefs." So he too had to strike out on a lonely path in the beginning, just as I have had to do. But later on, after he had proved his thesis, he acquired professional help.

In closing this chapter, I want to pay tribute to another wonderful product—aloe vera—the use of which is spreading rapidly. It has been used as a healing agent for centuries by North American Indians, and is now catching on with other Americans.

A few years ago, the *Mother Earth News* magazine gave a report on a lady who had developed arthritis in her hands. She said her fingers stayed so swollen and stiff she couldn't make a fist. Her doctors tried every remedy from aspirin to gold, but her ailment kept getting worse despite the best professional care.

Then she recalled a childhood memory when she had lived in the Southwest. One of her Mexican neighbors had claimed that a person could heal a great number of ailments with the juicy pulp of the aloe vera plant. So she started drinking teaspoons of extracted aloe juice and rubbed her hands twice daily with the gel from a broken leaf.

It wasn't long before most of the swelling and stiffness in her joints went away, so she could even wear her wedding ring again. She reports that as long as she continues to use aloe vera—no more arthritic pains.

I believe in aloe vera very much. I used to use a great deal of it in my practice. I drank a glass of water with one teaspoon of aloe vera two to three times a day, with excellent results. I heartily recommend it to you.

The question posed at the beginning of this chapter was, do we need supplements? Let me answer it this way. Only in extreme situations, and then, only with moderate use. I firmly believe that chemical shortages in the body can be far better supplemented by natural foods, grown organically, and a change in lifestyle, exercise and positive mental attitude, than by drugs or supplements—and at far less cost.

Practically everybody in America has had some rheumatic or joint problems in their life. The current calcium craze is not needed if we balance our diet with the proper amount of sodium foods. Taking drugs for relief of acids and pains is only a temporary relief. They cure nothing. What we take in supplements we can get in foods—providing they are organically raised.

I believe at least 50% of the rheumatism in America could and should be taken care of with nutrition. When you get to rheumatoid arthritis and osteoporosis, perhaps 30% to 35% could be helped.

In the next chapter, I will cover the very controversial subject of vegetarianism and see what we come up with.

7

Vegetarianism—Right or Wrong?

There are many vegetarians who are not getting the proper development of lecithin in the body. Lecithin dissolves any hard material in the body. It also dissolves high calcium deposits. It goes to the aorta to dissolve the hard material that might have been stored there by having fried foods in the past. This is something we have to compensate for.

Fried foods or heated oils should never be found in the kitchen. They add to your joint troubles, causing a hard condition in the body and lowering of circulation to your extremities, where a lot of arthritis trouble may be settled. So, lecithin is very important to have in your diet.

Vegetarians do not get much of this element, and they have to supplement their diet. Vegetarians can control arthritis very well, if they become mentally good vegetarians. Harmful acids develop from resentment, resistance, hate, fear, overzealousness, jealousy; all of these negative emotions produce a breakdown of the mental parts of our being and finally create acids that rob the body of the sodium that is stored there.

Lecithin has to be returned to the body. It is a brain and nerve food. It is necessary for balance in the body, especially so as we get a little bit older.

Now, this takes care of some of the supplements that should be ingested by the body. I think I mentioned this before, but if not, let me comment on the fact that a veal joint has no meat on it whatsoever. We are cooking the material out of the ends of the joint bones. If you stop to think about it, when you throw a bone to your dog, you notice he always chews on the ends of the bone. He knows where the greatest food value is.

As far as sodium is concerned, it was covered in an earlier chapter. I will now discuss calcium. Calcium is found highest in seeds and nuts. It is also found in cheese. If you eat cheese, you should consume a *minimum* amount. Pasteurized cheese is all right if it is aged. Raw goat milk cheese is the finest of all.

Milk Products

As far as milk products are concerned, I suggest you use them sparingly. You can use kefir occasionally or milk that is made into a clabbered form or yogurt. But I must warm you that the commercialized yogurt does not balance the body well from a calcium standpoint. Experiments on some 29 rats showed that using the commercial yogurt, all ended up with cataracts. This is a sign of calcium out of solution.

First of all, that isn't a healthy diet and it could cause you no end of trouble. I believe the commercial yogurt is something that is not going to keep up a good calcium content in the body. If you do use that yogurt, always have other foods to offset it. The dried fruits and fresh fruits with yogurt are always a good combination.

You will find that all the old people who never had any joint problems seldom used fresh milk. It is always made into yogurt or clabbered milk, called matzoni in Russia or kumiss in turkey. This kind of milk can be digested very easily and quickly.

I have found practically everybody past the age of 45 lacks hydrochloric acid. Now if we are lacking it as we get older,we should be using only the clabbered milk instead of the fresh, because clabbered milk has been prepared the same way that hydrochloric acid would prepare it.

So, when you take clabbered milk, it is ready to be absorbed in the stomach and taken into the body without that amount of hydrochloric acid or enzyme we need to break it into clabbered milk. This is an important point, and I believe it is one of the longevity secrets of the old men and women.

The Importance of Whey

In addition, I have found that nearly all the old people were consuming whey, the residue formed from clabbered milk. This is called the old man's drink, and I do believe this kept their joints limber, as well as those of the older women. Whenever they made clabbered milk, they always had the whey. If you don't like the taste of it you can add a little honey or fruit or vegetable juices with it. Or you can find some way of flavoring it so it is easy to take.

I feel it is important to take digestive enzymes with each meal. I believe we should also take something as a supplement for the bowel. Five or six alfalfa tablets with each meal are necessary. Crack them before swallowing. You will find they help the bowel activity.

We should also take two teaspoons of psyllium husks in cereal every morning or you may use ground flaxseed meal instead. These will provide bulk and keep the lower bowel material moving along, and keep it softer. And for goodness sake, answer the bowel call. When nature calls, go to the bathroom. It is very necessary. I hate to tell this on myself, but once when I was having an interview with the King of Hunza, I had to excuse myself and rush to the nearest bathroom! That's how important I consider answering nature's call.

This reminds me of an amusing story about one of my sons when he was young. We always sent him to school with a nice sack lunch. With his sandwiches, we always included snacks of celery stuffed with fillings, such as chopped dates and nut butter. The sandwich itself always had leaf lettuce, and sometimes sprouts, cucumber slices and other vegetables. So there were vegetable fillings in the snacks and vegetable snacks to eat along with it, such as bell pepper slices, carrots, etc. We taught our children that when we eat bread, we must have vegetables with it. This would keep us from being constipated.

Once I asked my son, "How are you getting along with your lunches?" He said, "All right, but they call me a rabbit at school because I have so many vegetables." And I replied, "Well, what do you say to that?" He said, "I tell them at least I'm not a constipated rabbit!"

A lot of people who have hemorrhoid problems have had them caused by a constriction and a tightened rectal anal muscle. By answering nature's call *promptly,* these problems can be alleviated, and eventually eliminated.

Many people have bleeding rectal conditions. Hemorrhoid preparations are among the greatest over-the-counter sellers in this country. It is indicative of the heavy amounts of rectal troubles nowadays. They even sell you rectal kits to tell whether you have cancer or not. A rectal examination is a routine part of the doctor's complete physical checkup for his patients. To take care of rectal problems, make sure that your bowel is in good working order.

A Potty Program for Adults

I consider the modern toilet one of the most abominable man-made inventions. It is completely unnatural and has caused a great deal of constipation. Wherever I traveled in primitive areas, I found the only toilet was a hole in the floor. Why?

The natural position that Mother Nature intended for man to defecate is to squat. This takes the pressure off of the bowel mechanism and enables you to move its contents easily. Even in so-called "civilized" countries, some restrooms have the same setup as in primitive areas. They provide bars along the walls so the elderly and infirm can support themselves.

Now I realize this would be extremely difficult for folks who have severe rheumatic, arthritic or osteoporotic conditions. So I have a solution to propose for them.

When you sit on a modern toilet, simply raise your hands above your head. This will help to overcome the prolapsus (the falling or sinking of an organ) that so many people suffer from because of their wrong way of living.

A prolapsus inhibits the moving of the material in the lower bowel especially, as well as interfering with the blood supply to the ovaries and uterine areas. By raising your hands above your head and keeping them there while eliminating, this will help remove some of the rectum pressure.

When you follow this technique, you will find that you will not press against the rectum when you move your bowel. You will not be *forcing* the toxic material out through the rectum, causing more rectal flaccidness, and you will not be pressing against the veins of the anal exit. It is an absolute necessity to keep your hands above your head while you are having a bowel movement.

If you cannot keep your hands straight above your head, attach a little rope to a side wall. While you are on the toilet, hold onto the rope and this will help keep your arms raised.

There are times when you have to have bowel movements away from home. Then keep your hands folded on top of your head, just as you do at home. This will help tremendously. I cannot begin to tell you how much good I have accomplished with just this one exercise.

"Gravity-Ptosis" (Gravitosis)

This is a term I have created. Ptosis means the same as prolapsus—the falling or sinking of an organ. Many people have a common disability called ptosis of the transverse colon, which simply means a camel's hump in reverse. Instead of being somewhat straight across and inclined slightly upward, the transverse colon hangs down in a U-shape. It presses against the lower organs and causes a lot of trouble.

One thing that brings on this condition is the sedentary lifestyle of so many people, sitting down at their jobs all day long. This makes you tired, fatigued. Gravity has gotten hold of you. Your internal organs have fallen or prolapsed. This is especially true when you have a lot of gas, a dry stool and maybe having only one bowel movement a day or even less than that.

If you have arthritis, and if you can't get the granulated lecithin, take 2 or 3 of the lecithin capsules a day as a supplement. Take the granulated lecithin in hot water, as a broth.

Find out if there are any particular organs in your body that are underactive. Are you fatigued? Have low blood pressure? If so, you should add an adrenal gland substance, one with each meal.

When your body is lazy or when you have had operations such as for tonsils and appendix, which are lymphatic organs, you have to go back and clean up the lymph system. Removing an organ isn't going to correct the condition causing that organ trouble. Cleaning or draining the lymph fluid is a needed correction. For this reason, it is good to take a lymph gland substance, one with each meal. This helps the lymph system to eliminate unwanted toxic materials.

Another very important thing is that we should consider the thyroid gland. I have learned that 95% of the poeple who come to me have a low metabolism and a lack of thyroid activity. This is something that has to be cared for.

While a drugless doctor cannot prescribe thyroid substance, I think this should be taken up with your doctor. I have found that many times while the thyroid may be considered low, to be considered normal, you will find it is on the low normal side. A little extra thyroid substance, like Armor's thyroid, will help tremendously. You must counsel with your doctor on this.

You may think I have digressed from the subject of this chapter, *Vegetarianism—Right or Wrong?*, but I really haven't. For everything

I have discussed so far is important, whether you are vegetarian or nonvegetarian.

I don't want to take sides in this red-hot controversy, but I will give you my ideas and let you make up your own mind. There are several varieties of vegetarians. First are the purists who will consume absolutely nothing of an animal origin, not even eggs or milk. They won't even wear a stitch of clothing made from animal sources, if they can possibly help it.

Then there are the lacto-vegetarians who eat no animal products such as meat, fowl or fish, but will consume eggs and milk.

Then we have the partial vegetarians who will very occasionally have a little meat, fowl or fish.

I am not attempting in this chapter to change either vegetarians or nonvegetarians, but to show that a proper balance of foods, according to our food laws, requires a certain amount of protein.

If you want to go the cleanest way in foods, without doubt, the vegetarian way is it. But there are some pitfalls along that way, and perhaps I can help you avoid them. Even a pure vegetarian must go by the food laws in my Health and Harmony Food Regimen to meet all the chemical needs of a healthy body.

In order to have a proper balance of foods, one of our food laws requires a certain amount of protein. This is where many vegetarians come a cropper. They don't get enough protein. As a result, they overeat to compensate for this hidden hunger and gorge themselves on starches, with inevitable problems.

A friend of mine tells me when he lived in Chicago in the first quarter of this century, there was a famous vegetarian restaurant owner who was a staunch advocate of that way of life. Imagine my friend's shocked surprise when he came upon this gentleman in a regular restaurant devouring a huge steak! It was a shock he never got over.

One of our food laws says we need 6 vegetables, 2 fruits, 1 starch and 1 protein every day. That protein is very important—not only for the building and repairing of tissue—but for the proper maintenance of the 20% acid and 80% alkaline ratio of nutrients in the bloodstream. This comes from another of our food laws. Whether you are vegetarian or not, *nutritional balance* must be part of your food program. And this is where so many vegetarians fall short.

The Most Perfect Land Protein

After fish, I consider eggs the perfect protein. Many people say they are high in cholesterol, which can cause hardening of the arteries, hardened fat settlements. Now eggs are indeed high in cholesterol, but what food contains the highest amount of lecithin? Egg yolk. God put the lecithin right next to the cholesterol because it is lecithin that breaks down and dissolves cholesterol to balance it in the bloodstream.

If you fry eggs, you ruin the lecithin, and all you've got left is cholesterol. If you fry or bake anything with oil or fat, you ruin the lecithin, leaving cholesterol-forming food. This is why we have to cook all foods with oils or fats in them at low temperatures, temperatures below the boiling point of water. Boiled or poached eggs are best.

There are experiments with prisoners who had 15 eggs a day for a solid year without raising their cholesterol. In Egypt, a man over a hundred years of age averaged 13 eggs a day for 30 years, and didn't have a cholesterol problem!

Without lecithin, the fats in eggs will form a hardened fat in the body and will be attracted to the arteries and settle there. This applies to all foods that have oils and fats in them. The high cholesterol is from the lack of lecithin destroyed with high heat. I am talking about all eggs—fertile or otherwise. The best eggs to use are fertile eggs, from chickens free to walk around and forage. We should have what we call "earth eggs." This is very important.

I consider eggs the most perfect of all foods, in part, because Dr. Alexis Carrel was able to keep a chicken heart alive for 29 years, feeding it egg yolk. That, to me, is a very, very wonderful experiment. You can't name another one concerning foods as valuable as that.

Another reason I consider eggs the perfect protein is that they have all eight essential amino acids in amounts needed by the human body.

Eggs and the Vegetarian Lifestyle

Eggs, especially the yolks, are a wonderful protein food for everyone, including the vegetarian. Many who have tried to go the "pure" vegetarian way have encountered problems with dizziness or dizzy spells, periods of weakness, difficulty in thinking, etc. When milk, eggs or both were added to the diet, these problems cleared up. Nuts and seeds are fine supplemental proteins, but it is very hard to get by with them as the main protein source. The same is true of the grains and legumes.

Nutrition experts say that eight essential amino acids are necessary for our nervous system, and especially for the brain. Some of these are found in foods with lecithin, which is also needed by the nerves and brain.

There is very little lecithin in vegetarian foods. You can find some in all the oils and fats, and you find it in soybeans. In fact, lecithin in the concentrated form often comes from soybeans. Most of us using lecithin are burning it out of our system through overworking the brain and nerves. And it is hard, from a vegetarian diet, to restore lecithin and the essential amino acids once they have been depleted in the body.

While we have very little of these essential amino acids in the vegetarian foods, the egg yolk has all eight essential amino acids and lecithin.

Now, of course, there are a lot of cults, a lot of religions, there are a lot of people and doctors who do not believe in the egg yolk. But I lived in Sri Aurobindo's ashram in India, where, at the beginning, they never believed in using eggs or milk. But now they have the largest herd of cows in all of India today. They also have the largest egg ranch in all of India. All the Olympic records won by India came from young people who lived in Sri Aurobindo's ashram. Vegetarianism without eggs or milk is extremely difficult for nutritional reasons, and also because the lifestyle of the vegetarian is different from those who eat more stimulating foods.

Another reason we need proteins, fats and lecithin is because they build and maintain the glands. And, as the saying goes, you are only as young as your glands.

I have now given you quite a few hints on vegetarianism versus non-vegetarianism. As I said in the beginning of this chapter, I leave it up to you to make up your own mind as to which course you wish to take. There is no question but what vegetarianism is an ideal way of life, but not everyone can follow it. You can't generalize. Each person has to make his own determination.

Climate and environment have a lot to do with it also. Take the Eskimos, for instance. They live entirely, or did before the white man invaded their land, on animal fat, largely blubber, and fish. They would laugh you right out of their igloos if you tried to convert them to vegetarianism.

Hjalmar Steffanson, the famous Arctic explorer, lived among them for over a year, and finally adapted to their nutrition program. In fact, when he returned to America, he and group of university students lived on *nothing but meat* for one year, and thrived on it, with no apparent untoward results.

So, there are arguments pro and con on both sides of the controversy. You have to be your own judge and jury, based on your own experience, and no one else's. You know your own body better than anybody else. Listen to it carefully and it will tell you what to do. Most vegetarians just give up meat and call themselves vegetarians. A good vegetarian should be a student vegetarian. He should know his food and above all, the variety of proteins he can eat without starving his body tissues.

I will discuss a very important subject in the next chapter—the five elimination channels of the body. Unless they function properly, health is impossible.

8

The 5 Elimination Channels

I would like to talk about the five elimination channels: the skin, kidneys, the bowel, bronchial tubes and lungs and the lymph. They each eliminate 2 pounds a day. If they are underactive in the least, and the metabolism and metabolic rate are low in each of these eliminative organs, you cannot be well.

Elimination is absolutely important in any disease, and above all things, we must take care of the bowel. The bowel is the most important of all. I have achieved more relief in arthritic and rheumatic conditions by taking care of the bowel alone than I have by any other means.

It would be beneficial for you to carefully study the program outlined in my book, *Tissue Cleansing Through Bowel Management,* which you can get from your health food store.

In taking care of the bowel, it needs progressive exercising, such as stated in Chapter 4. In particular, the slant board is used for getting rid of the pocketed bowel condition, also covered in Chapter 4. This will give you a good start to compensate for the condition you may have developed over a period of years.

The most important and necessary chemical elements in the bowel wall are potassium, sodium, magnesium and calcium. You will get these chemical elements by following my diet and the supplements I suggested earlier.

For a healthy skin, I have suggested a daily skin brushing program, plus outdoor exercise and perspiration. If you will take one or two teaspoons of rice polishings daily, this will also help. The skin is a silicon organ. I find most people are lacking in this element. I have never yet found a person who has a good skin, so let's feed and care for that valuable part of the elimination system.

When it comes to the next eliminative channel—the lung structure—brisk walking takes care of that organ. I also suggest a sniff breathing program when you have poor oxygenation. When the thyroid is low, oxygenation cannot take place well. If you haven't been doing sufficient exercising in the past so there has not been a good exchange of oxygen and carbon dioxide, such as living in cities and working in offices where the air is polluted, you have to somehow get rid of that pollution overload.

I suggest you go out into the country as often as possible, where you can inhale fresh air and do the sniff breathing program outlined here. Sniff breathing exercises are done while walking in sets of 7 steps. The first 3 steps, take a third of a whole breath each step until the lungs are full at the end of the third step. On the fourth step, exhale fully through the nose by sniffing it out. The next 3 steps, don't breathe in or out, and start all over with the next step. Do 7 repetitions of the 7 steps morning and evening for two months, or until you have good chest activity.

It is necessary to do some deep breathing. By doing so, you will develop a good lung structure. That will help to eliminate all the catarrh, phlegm and mucus that you possibly can from what has been produced in years past.

You will find that the heavy catarrh will be gradually eliminated, getting less and less as you start cutting down on milk, wheat and sugar consumption. These are the three chief catarrhal producers in the body, and they wear down the lung structure, especially if inherently weak.

This is one of the reasons so many people develop pneumonia. Pneumonia is an extreme catarrhal condition that should be diagnosed and treated by a doctor. Lung congestion and pneumonia may be associated with heart trouble or with kidney problems. So you see that the lungs are a very important elimination channel to take care of.

Nothing Wrong With My Lungs

I treated a man a short time ago whose first analysis showed he had lung troubles. But he said, "I have nothing wrong with my lung structure." Four days later, he was in the hospital with pneumonia. He already had the problem beginning there. He already had a heavy catarrhal condition existing, and he found out it just took a little extra breeze, cold air, damp air, a little extra activity, overwork fatigue—all breaking down his body—and he landed in the hospital.

Many people are on the verge of getting a lot of these problems today. I might just mention that one study showed that six out of ten people who say they are feeling good or well have a chronic disease in their bodies. I believe this. But it isn't known how all of these chronic diseases are developing or from whence they came. I am giving you some very good hints in this book so you can work towards the *prevention* of disease and the overcoming of what you may have with any troubles at the present time.

It is a truism that whatever will prevent a disease will cure a disease. So now you have an opportunity to adopt a dieting program, a maintenance diet, a maintenance way of eating—supplements, exercises and so on.

Sometimes professional treatments are necessary. You got into a problem, and treatments of many kinds are fine today. Reflexology and kinesiology (muscle testing), touch systems and the reflex work I use are all good. But without a proper health harmony program of eating, it is all going to be in vain—and very costly.

I say this because we are living now in a relief society. Our healing programs, by and large, whether in the wholistic healing art or in the medical art, are to give you relief from your pain. The moment you get relief from your pain and find you can still walk, crawl, speak or navigate, you feel then that you are going to go on. You don't do anything to help yourself before you are in trouble. And this comes back to the idea that we deserve what we get. We get what we build up in our bodies.

My mother told me that you can have anything you want, son, but you have to take everything that goes with it. If you take enough coffee and donuts, you will follow up with a laxative. If you take enough pasteurized foods, an overabundance of oils that have been cooked and heated in the kitchen, you are going to have to take some treatments of some kind in the future.

Most of the treatments today are only given through our relief societies. If you want to correct these conditions and build new tissue in place of the old, the best way you can do it is to follow through with my suggested diet program. And especially for rheumatism, arthritis, osteoporosis, disk problems, etc.

Usually you do need supervision, but in this supervision, go more for correction. Don't just go for feeling good again now that you no longer have your disk problem. How about your bowel? How about the rest of your body? Is it *all* in good condition? What about the kidneys?

One of the best things to take care of the kidneys is to cut out all citrus fruits from your diet, unless it is completely *ripe*! Lean toward the vegetable kingdom instead of using too much of the fruit, which stirs up the body's acids.

An excellent herb for the kidneys is to take a cup of kidney-bladder tea or KB-11 tea, which you can get at your health food store. You can also use a kidney substance, taking one tablespoon with one or two meals a day.

The skin perspiration is going to help the kidneys. The skin is your third kidney, and as you work the kidneys properly, it is going to help their function. Also, corrective exercises will help the kidneys, as well as cutting down on meat, especially red meat.

We can sometimes overconsume liquids, which puts an overload on the kidneys. You can have a greater amount of fluids going into the body, but if you have a lack of fluids when you have a lot of metabolic breakdown products in the body, acids that are broken down in the body from dying tissues, you must make sure to take more fluids.

If you have hardening in the arteries or osteoarthritis, for example, I believe you should use distilled water for a while, that is, six months to a year. After that, use the reverse osmosis water. I suggest starting out with distilled water in extreme cases where the calcium has settled in the body and hardness has developed. Then start using ordinary water from reverse osmosis or good mountain water. Fresh, clean water is very necessary to keep the kidney elimination channel working properly.

Also there are side effects from drugs, which are very necessary to take care of. The residues of drugs are usually eliminated through the kidneys or through catarrhal discharges. So you want to make sure you have enough water to eliminate the residues of drugs and foods that our bodies cannot use. Taking two or three glasses of liquids before breakfast is the best way to flush out the toxins from the kidney and bladder. One of these glasses should have a teaspoon of liquid chlorophyll in it.

One final thought I have is that many people have come to me who have had arthritis, rheumatism, osteoporosis, bone and joint problems of any kind, and have lived on so many treatments in the past, all the way from gold shots, allergy shots, drugs, vaccinations, to using calcium-dissolving chelation, that I feel the side effects haven't been taken care of properly. This must be done.

Now, a few remarks on the last of the eliminative channels—the lymph system. A very important system, and one which has up to now been given scant notice in wholistic circles. One of its main functions is to return the blood proteins, the albumins, globulins and fibrinogens to the bloodstream. The protein molecules diffuse out of the blood capillaries, are picked up by the lymph capillaries, and are returned to the bloodstream by way of the lymphatic ducts. Impaired or inadequate drainage causes proteins and interstitial fluid to accumulate in the tissues, which eventually become swollen and painful. The lymphatic system also transports the long-chain fatty acids from the intestines to the bloodstream. Cholesterol is carried to the bloodstream mainly by the lymphatic system. Certain hormones and enzymes are believed to be transported in the lymph.

One of my former students, a very talented doctor, calls the lymph system "a garbage disposal system," an accurate description, I believe. If you will follow the suggestions I have given to keep all the other eliminative channels open and functioning properly, you will find it will also take care of the lymph system.

The day is coming soon when we will find out the condition of the various tissues in the body. We will then be able to see whether the tissue is inherently weak, whether it is toxin laden and whether that tissue has the proper chemical balance of elements so it can function the way it should.

When these things have been put together, then you will find that the doctor can furnish you with the outlines, with the program, with the correct lifestyle, with a balanced food program that you will need in order to put new tissue in place of the old.

This is sadly neglected in our diagnosing today. It is sadly neglected in our analyzation programs. We have malpractice insurance for those professionals who do the wrong things; who cut out an ovary, possibly, that shouldn't have been removed; for all the side effects that are being treated today; for all of the conditions that are given the wrong operation.

But we see that very little is being done to compensate for neglecting to put people on the right program, neglecting to tell them how to change their programs. Teaching is so necessary, and I don't believe a doctor should practice without teaching his patients how to live properly. This is particularly necessary with regard to foods and nutrition, giving the proper program to follow through every day.

Our Polluted Environment

Our doctor program is neglected, and it should be brought out to the front that we must take care of our public water supplies better. The pollution in our air and our foods, as well as the additives, should be diminished. There is so much that a doctor should be doing outside of treating in order to get people well and to keep them well. Here is where the greatest medical disaster exists.

Please understand that what has been suggested here does not mean you should take the place of your doctor in supervising your own health. A good doctor is a gem in your life. He can be the most valuable person in your family's health. You should consider him in utilizing the very finest treatment you can get. But you must always remember that there can be many alternatives that exist whenever we are using drugs. There are also many treatments that are not natural and proper alternatives, treatments that will not help to build a new body in place of the old one.

Glandular Disturbances

There has been so much talk about using estrogen as a supplement or as a doctor's prescription. We recognize that the glands themselves keep a great balance in the body, and are especially helpful in preventing sickness and problems that have to do with calcium and sodium metabolism. The glands often have been broken down in many ways, and I want to bring out the fact that when one organ goes bad in the body, it affects every other organ as well. If one organ is toxic and underactive, it can be a drag on the effective function of every other organ in the body.

It is not an unusual thing to have glandular disturbances these days. Many of them come from the fact that we do not have the whole grain foods and the seed foods that we should have in our diet. We have mostly cooked foods, which contribute to the toxins that have created our problem that we consider a disease today.

It has taken many years to develop, and I ask, "Where was the doctor in the beginning?" Now the "doctor" in the beginning should be in the amount of vitamin E that we have in all of our foods, and which has been destroyed in processing. It is vitamin E and lecithin that are destroyed in our foods by cooking, and also eliminated in our refining processes at the mill. All of our fast foods and pastries today have been vitiated, along with our flours that have been so refined that we have knocked out the vitamin E entirely.

Vitamin E is really a wonderful gland food. Our glands have become depleted in many ways from the foods that we now have. Your skin is as young as your glands. You find that when the glands aren't working right, they can affect every other part of the body. They can be the beginning of allergies, they can be the beginning of catarrhal problems, they can develop menstrual disorders. We see it in the different types of births we have today.

First of all, our birth control methods are causing a lot of disturbances. They deprive us of the proper chemicals. The myriad number of drugs we consume today that settle in the glands themselves are causing thyroid troubles, pituitary gland troubles, adrenal gland troubles, and so many problems with the glands that it is almost unbelievable.

Our refined food products cannot build a good pancreas, they cannot build any glands that are good in the body. We resort a good deal to estrogen, Premarin, etc., in order to get these glands to work proprly. But we promote a stimulation without taking care of the rest of the body. The body needs a good glandular system in order to have it function well.

The Wholistic System

We have to look at the body from a wholistic standpoint. To expect estrogen to control the calcium in the body and to be taking that alone for osteoporosis, as an example, is a sign of neglect, because we are not taking care of the rest of the body. The eliminative organs haven't been treated properly in many cases. The liver also must be taken care of as well. We have to realize that the body is a whole unit, not simply an aggregation of many parts, each part to be treated separately by suppressing symptoms of discomfort.

Estrogen is for glandular problems, but is also classified as a drug in its side effects. It is being hotly argued whether or not it causes cancer. If there is any doubt whether it is, we should be using an alternative that doesn't cause cancer.

To make up for our past where we haven't had the foods that are proper, we should zero right in at the kitchen and make sure that we don't have heated or too many concentrated oils. We should make sure that the nuts and seeds we use are raw. This will compensate for the nuts and seeds in the past that we have roasted or used in baking. They were usually salted and had the oils and fats heated so they were not proper foods. The law of compensation comes in here, and we have to, many times, resort to glandular extracts and glandular foods to make up for our deficiencies.

I feel that we should try to use the alternatives first. In my teaching and lifestyle habits, this is the most important I always considered.

To sum up, making sure all five of our eliminative channels: the skin, kidneys, bowel, bronchial tubes and lungs and the lymph system, are working efficiently will do more for the body than myriads of treatments.

As one of the TV ads says, "It's so simple. Get back into life!" It is really very easy, and very inexpensive.

In the next chapter, I will tread on those coals of fire called sex problems. There is nothing more controversial, and I hope I come through the ordeal unscathed!

9

Is Sex Necessary?

For those who believe sex is for the propagation of the species, the answer is yes. For those who don't care about the propagation of the species, the answer is no, but it is is desirable. I guess we all fall somewhere in between these two extremes.

Whatever our individual belief, sex, indeed, has a lot to do with the estrogen values that the female needs and the androgen values a man needs. I feel that the sex life is one that should be normal. But what is "normal"? There is no such thing as "normal" that is good for everybody.

I don't know whether celibacy is the answer for a lot of sexual problems, but I know a lot of people are not going to be interested and won't follow that practice.

Celibacy belongs to a certain kind of person. It belongs to the one who wants to give up his/her life and his/her energies to live possibly the extreme vegetarian life, wants to become a monk, a nun, or wants to lead a certain type of life of service to his fellowmen. There are indeed people who want to do that, and I think it is perfectly all right, if it is according to their calling and lifestyle. Each person is made up of different physical, mental and spiritual material. We thus have to consider it "normal" for them.

But for those who do not consider that path as their lifestyle and are getting into an active sex life, we have to remember, first of all, that a normal sex life keeps us away from frustration. Frustration can burn out the chemical elements in the body. Those who live in hate, jealousy and fear upset the glandular system more than anything I can tell you.

It cannot be said that you have sex once a week, once a month or whenever you do have it. Some people have a high drive. Having a low drive, when the partner has a high one, may be caused by not getting together in the emotional outlets. This emotional outlet can be a happy moment in life and can be helpful to the arthritic person, because the emotional life that comes from sexual frustration can cause a lot of trouble with arthritis, rheumatism and osteoporosis.

There is a certain amount of stimulation that comes from the sex life. Some of that stimulation can never be exercised in any other way. It can be a helpful and corrective feature for the body.

I do not believe that the sex life can be a determinant in ending our life, unless we abuse it. There is what is called a biological urge. There is a magnetic attraction. This is what we call a "turn-on" in one person for the other. If these urges aren't answered by being taken care of and corrected, many times our body has to adjust to these mental attitudes to the proper sex life, and what follows when we do not have it.

In many people, his or her sex expression follows the other one in the married life. It can be adjusted and can be followed very well, in many cases. But when it is not taken care of, we should seek a solution. Solutions can be found in proper diet, in exercise programs, in a healthy mental program, spiritual practices and professional counseling.

Many times our occupation can interfere with our sexual life. In the long run, it can interfere with our balance and metabolism that are so necessary for having a good equilibrium in any one of the diseases that can develop in the body.

To be cared for and to be loved is part of a good sex life. To be cared for and loved is also part of a "no sex" life. And it has been discovered that deficiency has to be cared for. To be turned on is one thing that may be physical. It can be strictly a glandular condition that we are reacting to from a physical standpoint. But when it is, when this turn-on comes physically, and it can be done with the proper feeling for another person, I believe it can help many illnesses.

Many people are going through life ragged mentally, and they are going ragged from a spiritual standpoint as well. It has to be looked to from a correction point of view.

There are many natural estrogens from a drugless aspect, and I do feel that using vitamin E is one of them. I also feel that taking a glandular supplement is, many times, necessary. If you are medically inclined, sometimes it can be prescribed only by adding the estrogen, Premarin, etc.

While I do not approve of using drugs, many people cannot do the work or accomplish the job through the drugless healing method. Then it is sometimes necessary that they resort to the use of drugs, which, in the long run, could produce side effects. What they will do, where they will end up, what organ will get the greatest brunt of the trouble, is hard to say. Usually they go to the weak organs in the body. They go to the inherent weaknesses in those organs that have had a lot of exposure in the past to drug residues, chemical additives in foods, air and water pollution, etc.

Taking care of our health is a full time job, and it requires a good doctor to see the whole program. To neglect looking at the body from a wholistic standpoint, creates dangers that we should not be subjected to.

Sun Chlorella

One of my latest and most exciting discoveries is Sun Chlorella. It is a product that any person can use very well. Sun Chlorella has just come on the market recently, and it is a big advancement over the chlorella in ordinary use. Why? Because the cell wall structure of this particular alga has been broken down so that it is now 48% more digestible than other chlorella, making this particular brand of chlorella one of the finest foods to take into your body.

According to the experiments that I know about, I have seen some great work done by Dr. Liang-Ping Lin in Taiwan, China. Some of the best work that he is doing is now being monitored at the University of Michigan. He has found that chlorella has an affinity for the drugs and heavy metals that have settled in the body. It is attracted to these elements, and it helps to move them out of the body.

The side effects many people are being treated for today could be eliminated if we could find the proper alternative. I feel that this is a great alternative and a great thing to be used in taking care of the whole body. Because it is sun-packed with sunshine energies, it has all of the elements that take care of arthritis and rheumatism problems, which is the sun energy.

There is no food, I believe, that is better controlled and developed so we can get the best health results, than the Sun Chlorella. It is a whole food, helping the whole body.

Bee Pollen

There is one other food that I think is valuable to take, and that is bee pollen. Some authorities believe it is an aphrodisiac, but I think that is debatable. I have had patients who used it with no such results. There are a few things to be said about bee pollen, and I do feel there have been a lot of useful experiments with it made on arthritis, rheumatism and osteoporosis. Some beneficial effects have been reported.

Now, if you take either one of these products without going on the proper diet, or just take one treatment from a doctor, that is not enough. We have to consider the whole body when we treat it. And while you may want to see results in a hurry, I can tell you that in most cases it takes a year's time to get the results you are seeking.

Don't be afraid to have a clinical diagnosis. Don't be afraid to have the whole body gone over with every test possible. Whatever you find wrong in any part of your body, it is to your advantage to take care of it. Every organ affects every other organ in the body, and that means from a good health standpoint. It also means from a toxic or disease standpoint. One underactive organ not getting the proper supply of blood or affected by poor circulation is going to affect every other organ in the body.

In having an examination, make sure that the elimination channels are tested. And, of course, the biggest problem in examinations today is that the doctor does not usually find out when you are in the beginning of problems that are yet to come. And this is something where many of the symptoms may be clouded over by suppressed catarrhal problems and drugs so that he does not see that you are on your way to future problems.

The body works as hard as it possibly can to keep you in good health. This is a natural function of the human body. It works for regeneration and rejuvenation as much as we allow it.

When we start developing creatinine (the end product of the metabolism of creatine, an amino acid present in tissues, particularly muscle), it is too late to consider how we got it in the beginning. When we finally develop low insulin and sugar imbalance in the body, something has been going on for some time. Most diabetics start taking insulin when they find they have sugar in the body. If we could discover these conditions long before they show up in our average test today, it would be a great boon to the healing profession.

The SMA Test

One of the tests we should be considering most, one of the tests I think is most useful, is what is called the SMA. This tests out some 20 different conditions in the body: sugar, chemical balance, mineral balance and a blood count. A urinalysis is also taken.

Fundamentally, this just tells what your body chemistry is doing so that possibly you know in what direction you need further help. But if we are the least bit anemic, if we are on the low functioning side, this is the time bring it to normal. Because any condition that is below normal is not good enough when you want to get well, especially if you have a chronic disease.

Many times we become chronically ill because of anemic conditions that show the blood count is just not up to what we call high normal. If you are going to get well, you want to be active normally, and above active in most cases, if you have a chronic disease in many organs in the body.

I feel that probably the best method of balancing the sex life and normalizing its emphasis in society is for each of us to develop a healthy, clean body. A healthy body is necessary to have a healthy mind, and a healthy mind puts the sex life in proper perspective. Sex is an important aspect of life, but it is far from the most important.

While I have covered the subjects of rheumatism, arthritis and osteoporosis in a general way, so far, I consider osteoporosis so important that I am devoting the next chapter to it. It has become a crisis for millions of women. Few men are afflicted. I consider it a totally unnecessary disease that can be nutritionally conquered.

10

The Scourge of Osteoporosis

It has been estimated that between 15 and 20 million Americans suffer from this disability—most of them women. Osteoporosis (porosity and weakening of the bones through calcium loss) is epidemic these days among women over 60, and common among younger women. Men may have it, although less commonly. Chemical changes in women's bodies after menopause make them more susceptible to this condition, but it can be prevented by proper diet and exercise.

Sometime between the ages of 50 and 65, the vertebrae begin to collapse under the body's weight. It is estimated that some 300,000 osteoporosis-related hip fractures occur annually and that more than 50,000 Americans will die from complications following hip surgery for hip fractures. This makes osteoporosis the 12th leading cause of death in the United States.

Of those who do survive, few will regain full mobility and some 100,000 elderly persons will seek care in nursing homes because of severe impairment from osteoporosis-related spine or hip fractures.

When you reach the age of 40, your ability to replace lost calcium declines. Because of this, nearly all of the elderly may exhibit some evidence of osteoporosis. While men are not immune, it is estimated that women suffer some eight times more from this scourge.

Women most likely to get osteoporosis are those who are thin, white, small-boned, those who get very little physical activity in their work and do not exercise. Those who smoke and have a family history of osteoporosis are more likely to get it than those who do not. The most dangerous time of life, as previously mentioned, is after menopause.

Densitometry

As a result of the multitude of osteoporosis sufferers, a new test has been devised, called densitometry. It measures the density of mineral content of a person's bones. It is considered an improvement over X-rays.

Two types of machines have been manufactured. Both measure bone density by penetrating the bone with a beam of radioactivity. They have caused a debate over which is the better method and the cheapest from a cost standpoint.

One is called a single photo densitometer. It uses a radioactive substance called iodine-125 to produce a single beam of radiation that measures the bone density in the forearm. The machine is portable and the test takes about 20 minutes.

The double photon densitometer uses two beams and a substance called gadolinium to measure bone density in a person's spine. The machine is too big to be moved readily and the test takes about 30 minutes.

An unidentified nuclear medicine specialist says that the radiation from both machines is negligible. But I find this an unacceptable opinion, for I don't believe *any* radioactive substance is good for the human body. I realize X-rays have become so well established as a routine in health work that they are seldom questioned. I believe they should be used only if absolutely necessary, and then at a very minimum.

About 10 or 15 years ago, a Tucson, Arizona, newspaper carried a full-page article on the sensational development of a new method of making X-rays at a Houston, Texas, hospital where the famous heart surgeon, Dr. Michael DeBakey, practiced. It was based on ultrasound, which gave a far superior and *three-dimensional* view of the body than ordinary X-rays. It was called holographic and was said to be completely nontoxic.

As far as I have been able to determine, not another word of this remarkable breakthrough has ever been printed. My guess is that had it been promoted, it would have destroyed the billions of dollars invested in standard X-ray equipment. The bottom line in all of these advances is still the almighty dollar.

You know that on our money we find the phrase, "In God we trust." But there is a typographical error there. It should read, "In *this* God we trust."

As I write this chapter, I have just seen a shot on TV of another similar device that I just described, some kind of a new holographic machine using ultrasound that gives a three-dimensional picture of the head and brain. So we will see what comes of this. Probably the same thing that happened to the previous device.

It is estimated that the annual cost of treating osteoporosis runs from $1 to $3.8 billion dollars. If just a small portion of this huge sum were spent on investigating wholistic methods, we wouldn't have to rely on sophisticated equipment to get results in the healing arts.

As I have maintained for years, the best time to start thinking about your health problems is early in your life, not when you become elderly. This makes it much more difficult to treat, but there is help even then. But not to the extent that would result from an early start.

Preventing Osteoporosis Through Correct Diet

Experts say that women should have at least 1,000 mg of calcium daily before menopause, and from 1,200 to 1,500 mg after menopause. Average consumption in U.S. women over 45 is 450 mg daily, according to studies. Dr. Morris Notelovitz, who has studied the problem, believes that an intake of 450 mg of calcium daily would result in a *net loss of 1.5% of bone per year.*

Among the best sources of calcium, I recommend yogurt, hard cheese, sardines, salmon, kale, collard greens, turnip greens, mustard greens, broccoli, seeds and nuts. I feel raw sesame seeds, sunflower seeds and pumpkin seeds are the best, while the almond is the king of the nuts. It is best to take the nuts and seeds in the form of nut and seed butters or nut and seed milk drinks. I do not recommend milk because I believe most Americans have too much of it, the pasteurized variety, that is. If you feel you must have it, the best is raw goat milk or raw cow milk made into yogurt or kefir.

Factors that hinder or block calcium assimilation include the oxalic acid foods (spinach, chard, cranberries, rhubarb), lack of vitamin D (the sunshine vitamin), overuse of protein, salt, coffee and alcohol. Frequent dieting can deplete calcium, as can soft drinks high in phosphorus. A high percentage of women with osteoporosis have a history of cigarette smoking.

The best calcium supplements, if not enough can be taken in foods, include bone meal in the diet. If not exposed to sunshine for at least half an hour a day, take a vitamin D supplement to assist in assimilation.

Because bones fracture so easily in those with advanced osteoporosis, thousands of deaths take place each year from the basic cause of weak bone structure. You may find the following chart helpful.

Calcium in Foods (mg/serving)

Low-fat yogurt (plain), 1 cup	410
Low-fat yogurt (w/fruit), 1 cup	318
Cheddar cheese, 1 oz	204
Swiss cheese, 1 oz	272
Tofu, 4 oz	154
Collard greens, 1 cup	355
Kale, 1 cup	206
Mustard greens, 1 cup	193
Sardines, 3 oz	372
Salmon (canned), 3 oz	285
Sesame seeds, 1 cup	165
Sunflower seeds, 1 cup	174
Turnip greens, 1 cup	269
Broccoli, 1 cup	136
Almonds (raw), 1 cup	332

The Need For Exercise

Exercise is extremely important in the assimilation of calcium. When astronauts are sent on space missions, they take calcium supplements with their food, and they exercise regularly, as much as the confines of their space suits and vehicles allow. But they nearly always return with a calcium deficiency, even if the space flight is only for a few days. The reason this happens is that exercise must be more than can be done in present space craft. We have to move the arms and legs to drive the blood. Walking and swimming are the best exercises, but neither can be done on a space craft.

In conclusion, let me assure you that if you will faithfully follow the suggestions I have given you in this book, you will get results that will surprise you. And at the lowest cost. However, if through lack of attention to proper dietary regimes or a faulty lifestyle you have reached an irreversible position, then you may have to resort to relief measures.

But, my fervent prayer is that you have not reached that drastic stage and that the principles outlined in this book will bring you far better health than you now have. I wish you the very best.

11

Daily Health Building Regimen

For those with arthritis and other chronic calcium-imbalance conditions, it is almost impossible to get well without following a proper diet and exercise program. We have to take care of the overacidity of the body. We have to restore calcium balance. We have to build new tissue in place of the old in all parts of the body where tissue has become underactive and possibly toxin laden. We have to let go of the old lifestyle habits and bad food habits, because we need to stop breaking down before we can start building up. These things can only be done right when we follow a definite daily regimen, and my many years of sanitarium experience have shown that the following regimen is very reliable and effective.

Carefully read the following rules and food laws and think about them. While these rules are ideal goals for the average person and may vary a little with the individual, start out by following them closely.

Rules of Eating

1. *Do not fry foods or use heated oils in cooking.* Frying lowers nutritional value, destroys lecithin needed to balance fats and makes food harder to digest. The temperature at which foods are fried or cooked in oil alters food chemistry, which is not a safe

practice. This can be one of the greatest contributing factors to cholesterol formation and hardening of the arteries and heart disease.

2. *If not entirely comfortable in mind and body, do not eat.* We don't digest food well when we are upset or when we are not comfortable. It's better to wait. A little waiting period from food will allow us to digest our food properly.

3. *Do not eat until you have a keen desire for the plainest food.* Too often, we eat simply because it is mealtime, not because we are hungry. Break this undesirable habit. To have the best possible digestion, eat when you are hungry.

4. *Do not eat beyond your needs.* Overeating is not good for the health.

5. *Be sure to thoroughly masticate your food.* Chewing well increases the efficiency of digestion. You get more food value for the money you spend on food.

6. *Miss meals if in pain, emotionally upset, not hungry, chilled, overheated or ill.* Each of these conditions is a signal that we need rest, warmth, calmness or something other than food which, if eaten, ties up considerable energy and blood in the gastrointestinal tract. Often, rest is the thing most needed. Food takes energy to digest and involves work by several organs, and it may take hours before food energy is available.

Rules For Getting Well

1. Learn to accept whatever decision is made. Do your best to keep your peace of mind. Peace is a healer.

2. Let the other person make a mistake and learn. This is so much better than standing over people and supervising every move. Learn to give the person the opportunity to grow and grow up. We are bound to make mistakes. Let's not gloat over them or live in remorse about them.

3. Learn to forgive and forget. Many studies have now shown that forgiving enhances health and helps prevent chemical changes in the body that may lead to disease.

4. Be thankful and bless people. These are two of the main secrets to a healthy life.

5. Live in harmony—even if it is good for you.

6. Don't talk about your misfortunes or illnesses. It doesn't do any good for you or the person you tell, and it presents an opportunity for them to do the same to you. Save it for your doctor. He's paid to listen to your troubles.

7. Don't gossip. Gossip that comes through the grapevine is usually sour grapes.

8. Spend 10 minutes a day meditating on how you can become a better person. Replace negative thoughts with positive ones.

9. Exercise daily. Keep your spine and joints limber, develop your abdominal muscles, expand your lungs—with specific exercises on a regular schedule.

10. Walk 10 minutes barefoot in the dewy grass or sand the first thing in the morning to stimulate the blood circulation.

11. No smoking or drinking of alcohol. Both nicotine and alcohol are depressant drugs. Both require energy to detoxify the body which is needed for more useful life processes.

12. Go to bed by 9 pm at the latest, when you can. If you are tired during the day, rest more. Rest allows the body to give its full attention and energy to healing and rebuilding tissues. Write down your problems at the end of the day and go over them first thing in the morning when you are refreshed, so you can look at them with a fresh mind and body.

Total Healing Laws

Food is for building health. You need to have foods that will meet the needs of a vital, active life and the following laws are designed to do exactly that.

When a person has joint troubles, it means that sodium has been depleted—not only from the joint areas—but also the walls of the gastrointestinal tract, where it is normally stored. Any rheumatoid condition is accompanied by poor digestion and assimilation, and by bowel troubles. It is especially important to follow the healing laws to bring back proper digestion and elimination as soon as possible. Also, anyone with an arthritic condition should seriously consider a bowel cleansing program, as described in my book *Tissue Cleansing Through Bowel Management.*

Work out your diet program to harmonize with the following food laws.

1. Food should be natural, whole and pure.

Reason: *The closer food is to its natural, God-created state, the higher its nutritional value.* Some foods, such as meat, potatoes, yams and grains must be cooked. Whole foods are more nutritious than refined, bleached or peeled foods. I'm not telling you to eat banana skins and avocado seeds, I'm just giving you a practical guideline. Pure foods are much better for us than foods with preservatives, artificial colors or flavors or chemical additives of any kind.

2. We should have 60% of our foods raw.

Reason: *I am not advising a raw diet because I like the taste, I'm saying it is better for us.* Raw foods provide more vitamins, minerals, enzymes, fiber and bulk, because they are "live" foods at the peak of nutritional value, if properly selected. Raw foods help the digestive system and bowel. I mean fruits, berries, vegetables, sprouts, nuts and seeds. We have to cook cereal grains, lima beans, artichokes and other foods, but there are many we can take raw.

3. We should have 6 vegetables, 2 fruits, 1 starch and 1 protein every day.

Reason: *Vegetables are high in fiber and minerals. Fruits are high in natural complex sugars and vitamins.* Starch is for energy and protein is for cell repairing and rebuilding, especially the brain and nerves. *This is a balanced combination of foods.*

4. ***Our foods should be 80% alkaline and 20% acid.***

Reason: *We find that 80% of the nutrients carried in the blood are alkaline and 20% are acid. To keep the blood the way it should be, 6 vegetables and 2 fruits make up that 80% alkaline foods we need, while 1 protein and 1 starch make up the 20% of acid foods.* To keep the blood balanced, we should eat 6 vegetables, 2 fruits, 1 starch and 1 protein daily.

5. ***Variety: Vary proteins, starches, vegetables and fruits from meal to meal and day to day.***

Reason: *Every organ of our body needs one chemical element more than others to keep healthy.* The thyroid needs iodine, the stomach needs sodium, the blood needs iron and so on. We also need variety in vitamins. The best way to take care of this is to have variety in our foods.

6. ***Eat moderately.***

Reason: *The healthiest people I have met in my world travels were the same weight later in life as when they were in their 20s, and some of them were over 120 years old!* In the U.S., 60% of the people are overweight, which leads to many health problems. Leave that extra food on the plate. Eating at home is more desirable. *The bigger the waistline—the shorter the lifeline.*

7. ***Combinations: Seperate starches and proteins.***

Reason: *Have your proteins and starches at different meals, not because they don't digest well together, but so you will be able to eat more fruits and vegetables each meal.* People tend to fill up on protein and starch, then neglect their vegetables. I want you to have a lot of vegetables with each meal for your health's sake, and when you are hungry, they taste wonderful.

8. ***Be careful about your drinking water.***

Reason: *Most public water systems are now highly chemicalized because ground water sources are increasingly polluted.* The fruit and vegetables in my Health and Harmony Food Regimen supply much of the water your body needs. If you use broths, juices, soups and herbal teas, they will take care of any remaining thirst during the day. If you are still thirsty, try cutting down or eliminating salt on your foods. Salt creates a thirst. Use vegetable or broth seasonings instead. I advise distilled water for those who have arthritis but we don't really need much drinking water on my Health and Harmony Food Regimen. Reverse osmosis water purification units provide the best water for household consumption.

9. Use low-heat, waterless cookware; cook with little or no water and do not overcook.

Reason: *High heat, boiling in water and exposure to air are the three greatest robbers of nutrients.* Low-heat stainless steel pots with lids that form a water seal are the most efficient means of cooking foods in such a way as to preserve the greatest nutritional value. For oven cooking, glass casserole dishes with lids are fine. I approve of crockpot cooking, because it offers another low-heat method.

10. If you use meat, poultry and fish, bake, broil or roast it—but have it no more than 3 times a week.

Reason: *Baking, broiling and roasting—while far from perfect cooking methods—are at least more acceptable in terms of preserving more nutritional value. Cook at lower heats for longer times to retain the most nutritional value.* Avoid pork and fatty meats and use only white fish with fins and scales. Salmon is permitted, even though it isn't a white meat. Fatty meats lead to obesity, heart trouble and so on. Beef is too aggravating to those with arthritis, and I do not recommend using it. Eating meat can produce excess uric acid and other irritating by-products, causing an unnecessary burden on the body.

11. Avoid having an excess of one or a few foods in the diet.

Reason: *An excess of one or a few foods may provide too much of certain food chemicals for the body to handle, causing irritation, inflammation or possible allergies.* The average American diet is 29% wheat, 25% milk and 9% sugar, all acid-forming foods which lead to and aggravate any rheumatic condition. Excess of a few foods usually means lack of variety in other foods, which leads to mineral deficiencies. See my new book *Vibrant Health From Your Kitchen* for more information on the harm done by using too much milk, wheat and sugar. Milk substitutes: seed and nut milk drinks. Wheat substitutes: brown rice, corn meal, rye and millet. Sugar substitues: honey, date sugar, fruit concentrates, maple syrup and dried fruit.

12. Don't neglect important foods.

Reason: *Our health is determined as much by what we don't eat as well as by what we eat, which can cause nutritional deficiencies that lead to a future disease.* If we neglect most vegetables, for example, we prevent our bodies from receiving needed chemical elements and enzymes. Lack of sufficient proteins, carbohydrates and fats—any or all—can cause disturbances in the body, as can lack of vitamins, minerals, lecithin, enzymes and trace elements.

Daily Regimen

Organize your meals to use the food laws and instructions properly. Here is an outline of what your daily food regimen should be like, and this will take care of the food laws—the law of variety, the law of proportions, the law of acid/alkaline balance, the law of 60% raw food and so forth.

You can have half your daily allowance of protein at breakfast and half at dinner; half of your starch at breakfast and half at lunch. Starches and proteins together help keep you from snacking and experiencing hunger between meals, but you shouldn't have so much that you don't have room for vegetables. Avoid citrus fruits, most of which are picked six weeks early and contains a green citric acid.

Breakfast

1/2 starch
1/2 protein
Health drink

10:30 am—Vegetable juice or broth

Lunch

3 vegetables (cooked, raw or salad)
1/2 starch
Health drink

3 pm—Fruit or fruit juice

Dinner

3 vegetables (cooked, raw or salad)
1/2 protein
Health drink

Before Breakfast

It is best to have a couple glasses of distilled or reverse osmosis water or a drink of some kind before breakfast. This cleanses the bladder and kidneys. I have found the practice of taking a teaspoon of liquid chlorophyll in a glass of water is one of the best things to start off the day. I avoid citrus juices in the morning, as they stir up acids. Remember citrus stirs up acids, while vegetable juices carry them off. Other juices you might have are natural, unsweetened fruit juice—grape, pineapple, prune, fig, apple or black cherry.

Before taking a shower or bath, brush the skin over the entire body with a long-handled, dry natural-bristle brush, such as those sold at most health food stores. Do not use a nylon bristle brush. Avoid brushing sensitive areas such as the face and breasts with rough bristles. A softer brush may be used, if you choose.

Afterward is a good time to exercise to music as described in the chapter on exercise. The mini-trampoline is very good. Swimming or brisk walking is also excellent.

If the hands are stiff, try exercising them under warm-to-hot water to reduce pain, whatever temperature is most comfortable.

A barefoot walk in sand or grass will stir the circulation. Kneipp baths, wading in knee-deep cold water and drying off in air, are also excellent. A good substitute for the Kneipp baths is to spray the legs from the ankles to thighs with a garden hose, then walk around until the legs dry. Circulation is impaired in most of those with arthritic conditions, and it must be restored to get rid of the condition. It is important to have some activity every day to improve circulation. Hawthorn berry tea should be taken once a day to help the circulation.

Breakfast

Fruit, one starch and a health drink (broth, soup, coffee substitute, buttermilk, raw milk, hawthorn berry tea, oat straw tea, alfa-mint tea, huckleberry tea, papaya tea, etc.) Dried, unsulphured fruits should be reconstituted. Fresh fruit such as melon, grapes, apricots, figs, pears, berries, apple slices (or baked apple) may be sprinkled with ground nuts, seeds or nut butter. Ground sesame seeds, flax seeds, sunflower seeds and almonds are good. Try to use fruit in season. If you have a cooked whole grain cereal, sprinkle ground nuts and seeds on top, add chopped dates, raisins, prunes, figs or other dried fruit for sweetening or use a little honey or maple syrup. A handful of steamed raisins in any cereal has been a favorite with our family. We can use Swiss muesli any time.

10:00 am

You may have your potato peeling broth or vital broth (1 cup) or a cup of herb tea or vegetable juice. Potato peeling broth or vital broth should be taken twice daily for the first month, then once daily for the next two months. Either one may be taken or you may change from one to the other. They may be used at meal times or between meals, as you prefer.

Lunch

Raw salad: tomatoes, lettuce (no iceberg), celery, cucumber, spinach leaves, sprouts (bean, alfalfa, radish, etc.), green pepper, avocado, parsley, watercress, endive, onion, garlic, cabbage, cauliflower, broccoli, etc., in any combination. Top with grated carrot, beet, parsnip, turnip—in any combination. sprinkle with ground nuts and seeds. Add a little grated cheese, if you like. One or two starches may be used, plus a health drink.

All high oxalic acids should be avoided by those with arthritic conditions or osteoporosis. Oxalic acid foods interfere with the absorption of calcium, and make the body more acidic, irritating the joints. High oxalic acid foods are more damaging when cooked. Avoid the following: rhubarb and cranberries (avoid at all times), gooseberries, Swiss chard, beet greens and spinach. Beet greens and spinach may be taken raw in salads, once in a while.

3:00 pm

Broth, herb tea or vegetable juices. A wonderful drink for rheumatic conditions is a combination of carrot, celery, parsley and beet juice. Use 1/2 cup carrot juice, 1/4 cup celery juice and 1/4 cup mixed parsley and beet juices. Cherry juice or concentrate in herb tea is good for rheumatic conditions.

Dinner

Protein, vegetable or fruit salad, one or two cooked vegetables (such as squash, artichoke, cauliflower, spinach, chard, Brussels sprouts, broccoli, etc.) and a health drink. If you had a large salad for lunch, have a small one for dinner and *vice versa.*

Desserts

I do not believe in desserts; however, we find occasionally many people have to have them, so here are some suggestions. Have a sliced apple, a raw fruit salad, a mixture of cut-up apples and steamed raisins with maple syrup. Mix plain gelatin with cherry juice and put a little whipped cream on top. Or why not have a banana, pear or apricot?

Preparing Whole Grain Cereals

The best way is to use a wide-mouth thermos. Put the cereal grain into the bottle, cover with boiling water, seal and let soak overnight. Make sure there is room for the cereal to expand without breaking the thermos. Exception: Cornmeal must always be added to cold water and brought to a boil in a pan first, or it lumps. When it has boiled, pour the mixture into a thermos, seal and leave overnight. Cereal can also be cooked in a double boiler.

Ground Nuts and Seeds

You can grind several types of nuts and seeds in advance and keep them in small jars or plastic containers in the refrigerator. Bring them out at mealtimes. You can sprinkle these on fruits, vegetables, salads, cereals, baked potato—almost any food. Nut and seed butters are good and can be added to soups, broths, salads and drinks to increase protein.

Other Supplements

You can add psyllium husks, wheat bran, wheat germ, oat bran, flaxseed meal, dulse or broth powder seasoning on many foods to add fiber, flavor and nutritional value. Herbs are a fine addition. There are many good supplements to help take care of hardening of the arteries and hardening of the joints put out by various companies. Dr. John Ellis has shown that several types of rheumatism may be greatly relieved by taking 100 mg vitamin B-6 daily. If the rheumatism is linked to B-6 deficiency, relief should come within 90 days.

Suggested Breakfast Menus

Reconstituted dried apricots
Muesli w/bananas and dates
Oat straw tea
Add eggs, if desired, or sliced peaches w/cottage cheese

Fresh figs
Cornmeal cereal
Shavegrass tea
Add eggs or nut butter or raw applesauce & blackberries

Reconstituted dried peaches
Millet cereal
Alfa-mint tea
Add eggs, cheese or nut butter or sliced nectarines and apple
Yogurt

Prunes or any reconstituted dried fruit
Brown rice with cinnamon and honey or reconstituted raisins
Oat straw tea
Grapefruit and kumquats
Poached eggs

Slices of fresh pineapple w/shredded coconut
Buckwheat cereal
Peppermint tea
Or baked apple, persimmons
Chopped raw almonds
Acidophilus milk

Cornmeal cereal
Reconstituted dried fruit
Dandelion coffee or herb tea

Cooked applesauce w/raisins
Rye grits
Shavegrass tea
Or cantaloupe and strawberries
Cottage cheese

Suggested Lunch Menus

Vegetable salad
Baby lima beans
Baked potato
Spearmint tea

Vegetable salad (with health mayonnaise)
Steamed asparagus
Very ripe bananas or steamed unpolished rice
Vegetable broth or herb tea

Raw salad plate w/sour cream dressing
Cooked green beans
Cornbread or baked hubbard squash
Sassafras tea

Salad with French dressing
Baked zucchini and okra
Corn on the cob
Ry-Krisp crackers
Buttermilk or herb tea

Salad
Baked green pepper stuffed w/eggplant and tomatoes
Baked potato and/or bran muffin
Carrot soup or herb tea

Salad
Steamed turnips and turnip greens
Baked yam
Catnip tea

Salad w/lemon and olive oil dressing
Steamed whole barley
Cream of celery soup
Steamed chard
Herb tea

Suggested Dinner Menus

Salad
Diced celery and carrots
Steamed spinach, waterless cooked
Puffy omelet, vegetable broth
Herb tea

Salad
Cooked beet tops
Meat or fish
Tomato sauce
Cauliflower
Comfrey tea

Cottage cheese, cheese stix
Apples, peaches, grapes, nuts
Apple concentrate cocktail

Salad
Steamed chard, baked eggplant
Poached fresh salmon
Persimmon whip (optional)
Alfa-mint tea

Salad
Yogurt and lemon dressing
Steamed mixed greens, beets
Tofu w/soy sauce
Leek soup, herb tea

Salad
Cooked string beans, baked summer squash
Carrot and cheese loaf
Cream of lentil soup or lemongrass tea
Fresh peach gelatin w/almond-nut cream

Salad
Diced carrots and peas, steamed
Tomato aspic
Roast leg of lamb w/mint sauce
Herb tea

Best Foods for Arthritic Conditions

Potato Peeling Broth
(High in potassium)

Take peelings, 1/4-inch thick, from two large potatoes and simmer in 3 cups of water for 15 minutes. Strain and drink broth only; 2 cups daily for one month, then 1 cup daily for the following 2 months.

Vital Broth
(High in potassium and sodium)

2 cups potato peelings
2 cups carrot tops
1/2 tsp vegetable broth powder
3 cups celery
2 cups celery tops
Medium onion, for flavor, as desired

Chop or grate vegetables and greens, add to 2 quarts of water, bring to a slow boil, simmer 20 minutes. Strain off broth and drink 2 cups each day. You may add a teaspoon to a tablespoon of rice polishings before cooking, or after straining, to enrich it with B vitamins and silicon.

Veal Joint Broth (Dr. Rocine's recommendation)
(High in sodium and potassium—a proto morphogen)

Buy a fresh, uncut veal joint and wash it in cold water. Put in a large cooking pot, cover half with water and add the following:

1-1/2 cups apple peelings
2 cups potato peelings
1/2 cup okra (or 1 tsp powdered okra)
1 stalk celery, chopped
1 large parsnip
1 onion
2 beets, grated
1/2 cup chopped parsley

Simmer ingredients 4-5 hours and strain off liquid, throwing solids away. Makes about 1-1/2 quarts of liquid. Have one cup hot and store rest in refrigerator.

Acid-Neutralizing Broth
(Arthritis tonic)

To one cup of hot water, add 1 tablespoon lecithin granules, 1 tablespoon Whex (goat whey) and 1 teaspoon vegetable broth powder. Powdered whey may be substituted for Whex, if necessary. (Whex is available from Mt. Capra Cheese, 279 S.W. 9th Street, Chehalis, WA 98532.)

Barley and Green Kale Soup
(High in calcium)

Soak 1/2 cup barley in 1 cup water overnight. Add 1 quart water, 2 stalks chopped celery, 1 chopped onion. Bring to boil and simmer 1 hour. Add finely chopped or ground fresh kale (frozen is acceptable if fresh is not available) and simmer 20 minutes more. Before serving, add parsley and a little butter or sour cream.

Note: Some people with calcium deposits in the joints mistakenly think they are getting too much calcium. This is not true. The calcium deposits in the joints are due to chemical imbalance, and calcium foods are still necessary in the diet.

Evenings

The evening should be calm and relatively quiet, with bedtime at 9:00 pm, if possible. Before retiring is an ideal time to enjoy a hobby, talk to your spouse or a friend or even take a nature walk (before dark). Avoid hectic or emotion-rousing activities, which contribute more acids to the body.

Supplements to Take

These are suggested amounts only. You should get assistance from a nutritionist for the correct amounts, variety and combination. Not all have to be taken each day. Those marked with an asterisk (*) should be considered for daily use.

- * Vitamin A-25,000-50,000 units daily for infection and inflammation.
- • Vitamin B-Complex — For nerve support.
- * Vitamin B-3 (Niacin) 150 mg after each meal for circulation to extremities. Used with favorable results on early arthritis experiments.
- * Vitamin B-6, 100 mg daily, as recommended by John Marion Ellis, M.D. (If considerable relief from pain not obtained in 90 days, discountinue.)
- * Vitamin C-1, 500 mg daily for cleansing and for the immune system.
- * Vitamin D (Cod Liver Oil — check label for Vitamin A content and adjust separate Vitamin A intake to remain under 50,000 units.)
- * Vitamin E-600 I.U. daily for the glands and heart support.
- * Magnesium, 150 mg tablet three times daily for calcium balance.
- • Zinc, 25 mg for glandular support and calcium metabolism.
- • Iron — if anemic, consider iron supplements.
- * Chlorophyll, 1 tsp. in glass of water any time during day.
- * Water, 2 glasses distilled or reverse osmosis water before breakfast.
- * Sun Chlorella, 6-8 tablets with each meal to aid detoxification and hasten tissue repair.
- * Alfalfa tablets, 5 with each meal, crack before swallowing, to improve bowel tone and fuction.
- * Digest Aid tablets, 2 with each meal to aid digestion.

* Dulse (or Kelp) — check label for suggested amount, iodine for thyroid to support the metabolism.
* Bone meal tablets, calcium/magnesium supplement.
* Lecithin, 1 tbsp. granules twice daily for brain and nerves.
- Pancreatin, 1 or 2 tablets each meal (if gas or bowel disturbance present.)
* Beet tablets, 2 each meal, natural laxative and liver cleanser.
* Whey (Whex-see p. 55) high in bio-organic sodium.
* Sesame seed or almond nut butter, 1 tbsp. daily for calcium.
* Broth powder seasoning (instead of table salt.)
- Psyllium husks (ground), flaxseed meal (ground) or wheat bran or oat bran, for bulk.
* Potato peeling broth (vital broth), 1 cup once or twice daily (p. 108).
* Acid-Neutralizing broth, 1 cup twice daily (p. 109).
* Hawthorn berry tea for circulation, once or twice daily.

* *These are suggested amounts only. You should get assistance from a nutritionist for the correct amounts, variety and combination for you, personally.*

12 . . . . . . Concluding Thoughts

By following my daily health-building plan in the previous chapter, all body systems and structures will gradually improve without undesirable side effects commonly associated with most drug treatments. Exercise aids in limbering the joints and moving the lymph fluid, which brings nutrient materials into joint-spaces and removes metabolic wastes.

Anyone who takes the path of pain relief in cases of arthritis, rheumatism or any joint problems must be very careful because they are on a dangerous path. No correction is taking place, in most cases. Temporary pain relief is the only result. Drug side effects may create future problems, and the condition of the disease may continue to worsen even while symptom-relieving drugs are being taken.

Symptoms such as aches, pains and stiffness are indications that the body is not in harmony. Something is wrong. Symptoms are a sign that something must be taken care of.

In all rheumatoid conditions, there is acid buildup. The stomach is not digesting proteins right. Digestion and assimilation are not good, and circulation of the blood may not be up to par. There may be heart, lung and glandular problems present to further complicate the picture.

The thyroid gland, which controls the blood level of calcium, also determines the metabolic rate of the whole body. If it is underactive, possibly due to iodine deficiency, not only is calcium out of balance in the body, but the functional performance of the whole body is lowered. Typically, if one endocrine gland is not working right (the thyroid in this case), the other endocrine glands attempt to compensate, throwing the whole glandular system out of balance. One deficiency in the diet can lead to many undesirable results.

Glandular imbalance may hasten osteoporosis, which in advanced cases in women may lead to dowager's hump. We find that as osteoporosis gradually progresses, the bone density in the spinal column (and other bones of the body) is reduced. Gravity and posture put more pressure on the front part of spinal vertebrae, causing them to be changed into a wedge-shaped. This gradual collapse of the front part of spinal vertebrae creates a curve in the spine at about the shoulder level, resulting in the hump commonly called the "dowager's hump condition and restoring the spine to its natural curvature.

Generally speaking, aches, pains, swelling, redness and feverish conditions may be triggered by many different kinds of internal disorders in the body. Hering's law tells us, "All disease starts from within and comes out." There is only one naturally corrective approach we can take, and that is to reverse the problem.

The Reversal Process

In the reversal process, we are going back over the track that brought on the problem in the first place, correcting and changing those processes and habits which have contributed to the problem.

This may require lifestyle changes. Most people develop certain life patterns based on how they respond to their jobs, marriage, money problems, home life, diet and recreation. Many persons have a mixture of good habits and bad habits, and these can develop a mental, spiritual and physical syndrome in the body. Poor food habits, for example, create mineral deficiencies. A bad marriage stirs up nerve acids. Staying up too late, too often, wears the body down and brings on chronic fatigue and more acidity. We may experience job aggravation. All these things depress the human spirit. So, we have to look again at our lifestyle. We may have to go back and correct some of the conditions that have developed as a result of how we have been living. Taking drugs to relieve symptoms is not going to solve the basic problem. In fact, drugs may worsen the orginal problem and create new ones as undesirable side effects appear with their own symptoms.

This book should be the best news in the world to you, because it teaches how to correct the problem. We are not interested in just relieving the pain. That's not enough. Before the effects of correction begin to appear, you may still have pain the first week or even the first month. But when it leaves, it won't come back, provided that you stick with a healthy lifestyle. My program in this book is designed to uplift every organ in your body through a healthy, harmonious lifestyle.

You Can Change Your Mind

It's time for you to get your mind on the right mental path. Think positive. Think "I can do it." It's time to touch the finer things in life. It's time to honestly confront your troubles, face them squarely in front of you, and ask what is the cause of the problem.

You need to recognize that the solution to your aches and pains is not going to be found over any drug store counter. Television ads for pain nostrums tell you they are for "temporary relief" only. They are not correcting anything.

Why shouldn't we start at the beginning? You have to be careful about producing nerve acids and overworked kidneys from a poor mental attitude. You can improve your blood circulation, but what good will it do if you are circulating coffee and donuts? We have to honestly evaluate what we can and what aspects of our lifestyle may be contributing to a disease. We find out that we are trying to find a way to enjoy a bad way of living. It just won't work.

Know Your Foods

One of the best things you can do for yourself is read my book *"Vibrant Health From Your Kitchen."* You must know how to use foods properly to stay healthy, and this book explains how to get into a balanced way of dealing with foods. We need to know the food laws—the law of variety, the law of excess and so forth. When we break the food laws, we get into trouble with our bodies.

Food will not correct your troubles overnight, but it will bring permanent correction over a period of time. Only food can build new tissue. Drugs do not build tissue. Replacing old tissue with new tissue is the way of correction, the way we bring in the reversal process, working to build better, healthier tissue from the inside out. You can't build good tissue with coffee and donuts. You should know that. You can only build good tissue with a balanced diet.

The Path of Correction

We seek the path of correction, not the paths of relief.

Aspirin is one of the most widely sold drugs in U.S. today. I knew a lady who brought a bottle of a thousand aspirins because they were on sale. She expected enough headaches to use them up. Can you see what crazy thinking habits we can get into?

It is criminal to think we are helping ourselves when we treat aches and pains with relief measures. This is called suppression. Suppression leads to chronic conditions over a period of time.

Most rheumatism, arthritis and osteoporosis started out as an insignificant rheumatic problem in the beginning. Perhaps a little excess acidity, brought on by sodium deficiency. Then, the aches and pains began. Instead of correcting the problem, system-suppressing drugs were used. These drugs only drove the problem deeper into the body. We develop a disease by living the kind of lifestyle that brings on that disease. We get rid of a disease by reversing the conditions that brought it on.

What will correct a disease will also prevent it, and those who have this wisdom to eat right, exercises right and live right seldom have to worry about taking care of a disease.

We may start with coffee and donuts, imbalanced eating habits. When this brings on catarrh, aches and pains, we graduate to the use of drugs and nostrums for symptom suppression, driving the cause of the problem deeper into the body. Fatigue comes easily. We grow more and more disabled. We can't move easily. There may be swelling, fevers, discharges from the body, skin disorders. This is the sort of process that marks the onset of chronic disease.

I want to give you fair warning. This is the way the body works. Every doctor knows that symptoms suppression through drugs will not bring better health tomorrow. We have to think in terms of the future—we have to look for a new day, a better day, a brighter tomorrow.

Here is the quote from *The Book of Health,* edited by Dr. Ernst L. Wynder, that I hope you can appreciate.

> Health, as defined by the World Health Organization, is "physical, mental, and social well-being, and not merely the absence of disease or infirmity." Such a definition implies the positive quality of physical fitness, which means the ability to carry out daily tasks with vigor and alertness, without undue fatigue and with ample reserve energy to enjoy active leisure pursuits, and the ability to respond to physical and emotional stress without an excessive increase in heart rate and blood pressure.

Summing Up

I just want you to spend some time learning to take care of yourself. You can't fool around taking short cuts in life. Three cups of coffee a day doesn't sound like much, but in a year that's over a thousand cups. We can't build a better life by abusing our bodies. That much is clear.

Low basal metabolism. Everyone who comes to me with joint troubles has low metabolism, indicating a hypoactive thyroid gland, with resulting lack of control of calcium. Circulation to the extremities is cut down, as part of the general reduction in activity level of all internal organs, calcium is imbalanced two ways—by inadequate thyroid control, and by inadequate circulation to the extremities.

Poor digestion. Ninety percent of my patients are deficient in hydrochloric acid, needed in the stomach to digest proteins. Since most calcium comes in proteins, a lack of hydrochloric acid robs the body of calcium.

Not enough sunshine. Insufficient exposure to sunshine cuts down the vitamin D needed for the assimilation of calcium. Wearing glasses (real glass lenses) or working in a glass-enclosed building cuts down the ultraviolet light needed. Poor assimilation of calcium is the result in both cases.

Hypocalcemia. Those sensitive to gluten in wheat and other grain products may develop intestinal irritation, malabsorption and hypocalcemia (inadequate assimilation of calcium). The extreme condition is celiac disease, defined by *Taber's Cyclopedic Medical Dictionary* as "Intestinal malabsorption characterized by diarrhea, malnutrition, bleeding tendency and hypocalcemia. TREATMENT: Gluten-free diet which may have to be continued for an indefinite period." The excessive use of wheat products is the U.S., which make up 29% of the average diet, is one reason why we have such problems with calcium imbalance in the body.

Acid foods. Poor food combinations, devitalized foods, demineralized foods and plain acid foods which make up such a large part of the average diet contribute to mineral imbalance.

Additives. Chemical additives in our food, water and air (pollutants) are conducive to chemical imbalance. Excess use of sugar and salt leads to calcium imbalance.

Four elimination channels. The bowel, kidneys, lungs and bronchials and skin are among the most neglected organs in the human body. Neglect and resulting underactivity can lead to toxic conditions that encourage joint problems.

Sweating. Sweating is normal. Everyone should sweat at least three times per week. It's a natural way of getting rid of toxic material—about 2 lb. per day through the skin. But excessive sweating drains the sodium reserves from the body. At that time, a person must replace it through organic food sources or become deficient. This can be the beginning of joint and stomach disturbances, because the main reservoirs of sodium in the body are in the joints and in the lining of the stomach.

Over 50% of the people in the U.S. have the preceding problems, and that is why we have so much trouble with rheumatism, arthritis and osteoporosis. We need to realize that these same problems lower the activity level of our immune systems, making us more vulnerable to any disease.

For the preceding reasons, we have to take the wholistic view when we take care of rheumatism, arthritis and osteoporosis. We have to raise the health level of every organ and body system, because all of them become affected by the conditions that brought on the joint problems and calcium imbalance. And, when we treat the whole body, we find that the joint problems and calcium imbalance are taken care of.

The human body is a fragile machine, an instrument of a million strings. When we play harshly on those strings, we produce acids. We must find out how to play this instrument harmoniously. We must learn how to live a life of joy, harmony and happiness. Then the body is happy in the spirit it carries.

Diet. Avoid or sharply cut down on red meat, milk, wheat, sugar, caffeine drinks, alcohol, and rich seafoods such aslobster, crab, scallops and clams. Potatoes, eggplant, tomatoes and peppers irritate arthritic conditions in some cases. Try cutting them out for a month and see how you feel. If you're better, avoid them completely. Increase consumption of vegetables, especially green salads, fresh fruit, and whole grains other than wheat. Use more raw nuts and seeds, such as almonds, sesame, sunflower and pumpkin seeds. Instead of red meat, have broiled, or roasted chicken (no fried foods of any kind), or fish such as salmon, cod, sardines and herring. A diet that has reportedly helped some consists of brown rice, vegetables and fish, with little or no salt added.

Supplements. Use a good multivitamin or consult a nutritionist. Your supplements should include vitamins B6, niacin, C, E and the minerals magnesium and zinc. Evening prirose oil is reported to have helped many with arthritis.

Lifestyle. Cut out alcohol, tobacco and as many drugs as possible (consult with your doctor). Exercise regularly but not excessively. Get adeguate rest and recreation. Try to work at a job that matches your gifts and talents, make your marriage as harmonious as possible and give up resting and resenting. As far as possible, live at peace with all men.

I am trying to show you the path to right way of living. The person who can see the value of this book from an exercise, diet, nutritional and complete wholistic standpoint—is the one who is going to prevent problems in the future.

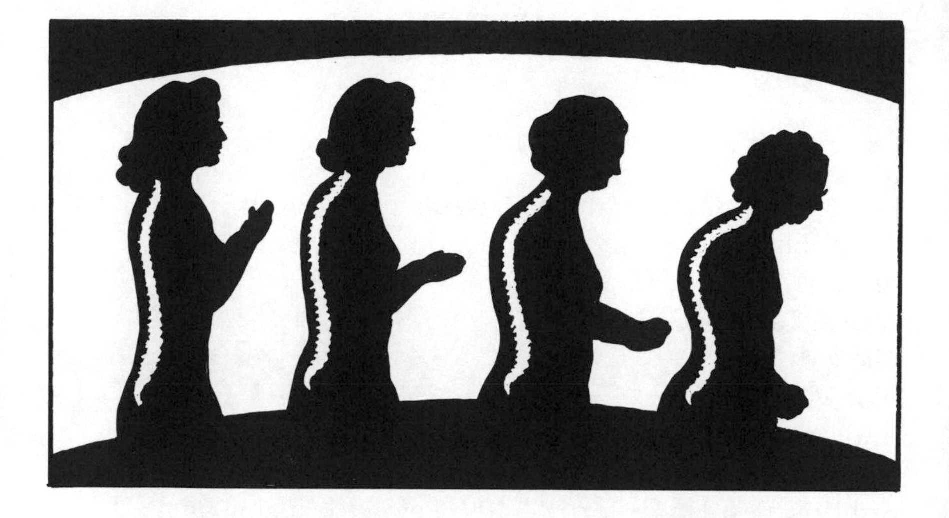

The "dowager's hump" develops as osteoporosis, gravity and posture combine to wear down the front of each spinal vertebra until it is wedge-shaped. The curvature of the spine is altered at the shoulders, as shown.

Index

C

D

I

J

K

L

M

R

S

T

U

V

W

For Your Good Health

Build a Library of Right Living—Look for Dr. Jensen's many books sharing the natural principles of happy, healthy living. If they are not available in your local bookstore or health food store, you may order direct from the address at the end of this ad.

THE WRITTEN WORD OF DR. JENSEN—His Best Books

Vibrant Health From Your Kitchen—Complete family food guide and nutritional teachings, with food laws, recipes and special new food remedies to keep the whole family healthy. Dr. Jensen says, "This is my greatest work for more abundant family health."

Slender Me Naturally—Want to lose weight safely, naturally and permanently? This wholistic approach to weight loss is geared to raise your health level as you take off the pounds you want to lose.

Nature Has A Remedy—Everything you always wanted to know about natural remedies, one of the most popular books ever written by Dr. Jensen.

A New Lifestyle for Health and Happiness—How to begin living a more natural lifestyle to prevent disease and enhance well-being in an age of fast living, stress and anxiety.

Creating A Magic Kitchen—How to turn your kitchen into a magic place where health and vitality flow into the entire family.

Tissue Cleansing Through Bowel Management—How to detoxify the body and keep it clean through diet and bowel management methods.

Dr. Jensen's "Man" Series

Food Healing for Man—A wonderful primer of nutrition and food facts for everyone, especially for those starting out in the nutrition field, exploring the role of deficiencies in disease and the restorative power of a balanced food regimen.

Chemistry of Man—The most neglected story in modern health care, the story of the chemical elements and their need in correctional nutrition for the prevention, reversal and healing of disease.

The Healing Mind of Man—Wholistic healing principles for the body, mind and spirit, including the roles of inspiration, wisdom, peace and beauty in healing. The many stories here from Dr. Jensen's experience will not only uplift but delight readers.

Published by
Bernard Jensen Enterprises
24360 Old Wagon Road
Escondido, California 92027

FOR YOUR GOOD HEALTH...

Start a Library of Right Living—Look for Dr. Jensen's many books explaining th natural ways of happy, healthy living. If they are not available in your local store yo may order them directly from the address below.

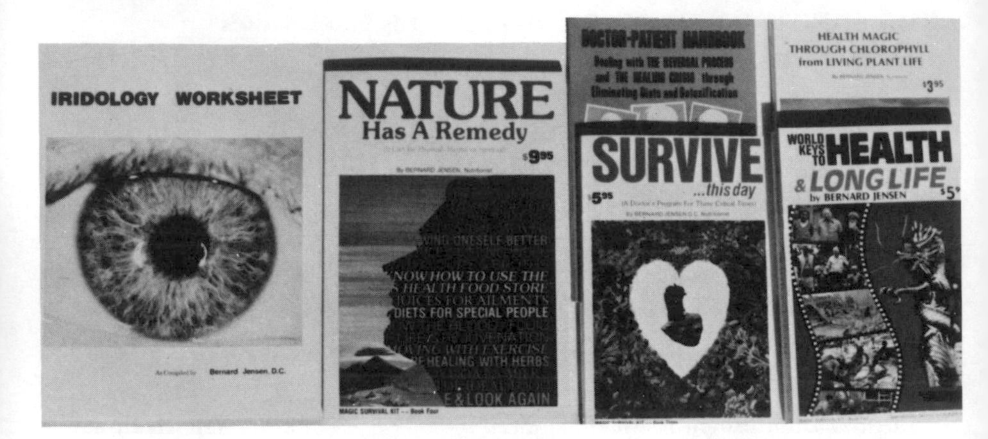

The *Iridology Worksheet* is a combination iris analysis workbook showing the findings of the analysis and a detailed explanation of those findings to be given to the patient. The worksheet portion is printed o NCR paper so that a copy is made automatically for your records. The booklet contains 16 pages, 8-1/2" 11".

A most valuable book, *Nature Has A Remedy*, is Dr. Jensen's practical remedies from his 50 years o sanitarium practice treating all types of ailments.

OTHER BOOKS BY DR. JENSEN

Science and Practice of Iridology
Iridology Simplified
Blending Magic
Creating a Magic Kitchen
Doctor-Patient Handbook
Joy of Living and How to Attain It
Tissue Cleansing through Bowel Management
Overcoming Arthritis/Rheumatism
Vital Foods for Total Health
You Can Feel Wonderful
You Can Master Disease
Health Magic through Chlorophyll
Survive this Day
World Keys to Health and Long Lif

SOON TO BE RELEASED

Arise and Shine, a spiritual treasury
Iridology Textbook, Volume II, practitioners' guidebook to the science.
The Greatest Story on Earth, how you are chemically put together.

Those interested may write for current prices on books and iridology supplies and for informatio on Dr. Jensen's Iridology Seminars-Internship Programs, Rejuvenation Seminars and the Ultimate Tissu Cleansing System practicum/instruction.